TOO STRONG TO GROW OLD

TOO STRONG

TO

GROW OLD

THE 40 AND OVER BEGINNERS GUIDE TO STRENGTH TRAINING TO STAY YOUNG, SLOW AGING, BURN FAT, AND LOOK GREAT.

PHILLIP J GERMANY II

JEROME-JOYCE AND ASSOCIATES PUBLISHING

Too Strong to Grow Old:
The 40 and Over Beginners Guide to Strength Training to Stay Young, Slow Aging,
Burn Fat, and Look Great.

Published by Jerome-Joyce and Associates Publishing LLC.

Book Cover by Ultrakhan22

Photos © Livia Productions.

ISBN-13: 9798649384155
    1.   Aging. 2. Longevity. 3. Strength Training. 4. Weight Loss. 5. Exercise.
    6. Health and Wellness. 7. Anti-Aging. I. Title.

Dedication

To God the father and his son, Christ our Lord, to whom none of this
this would have been possible.

To my wonderful family

Table of Contents

Acknowledgements

This book has been years in the making, but has finally come to fruition. It's been a long journey with the help of many people. Thank You.

TOO STRONG TO GROW OLD

Disclaimer

The information contained in the book does not constitute medical advice. The author is not a medical professional. This book is intended nor should not be understood as cure for any type of chronic illness, physiological, or psychological problem. Information regarding training regimens, movements, and nutrition are presented for information purposes only and may not be suitable to every individual.

The author and publisher are not responsible in any manner for any programs or opinions expressed herein. If you suffer from any health problem requiring medical treatment, it is advisable to consult your physician before taking any dietary supplement or embarking on any physical training regimen.

The author and publisher specifically disclaim all responsibility for any liability, loss, or risk, personal or otherwise that is incurred as a consequence, directly or indirectly of the use and application of any of the contents of this publication.

INTRODUCTION

"Do not, then, train youth to learning by force and
harshness; but direct them to it what amuses their minds,
so that you may be the better able to discover with
accuracy the peculiar bent if the genius of each."
- Plato

Phillip J Germany II

2

Are you 40 years of age or older? Are you tired? I don't mean out of breath or tired from lack of sleep or working all day. I mean tired of feeling drained, dragging yourself around, lethargic, no energy, no drive. Are you afraid that you'll never feel better and that this is the way you're supposed to feel at your age?

> Imagine eating what you want, within reason, and still look and feel great.

> Imagine burning hundreds of calories all day even when you're asleep.

> Imagine excelling at all of your activities and feeling good doing them.

Now imagine you have a bank account where you make regular deposits in a savings account and through the miracle of compound interest the amount grows. When you take money out or use some it you don't worry about the balance because you regularly replenish it and there is so much in account that a withdraw is not a big deal.

Now image your account with little money. You haven't been diligent in making regular deposits and when you go to make a withdrawal you have very little if anything in your account to work with.

Your body is the same way. Every time you exercise, strength train, and build muscle you're making deposits to your physical and emotional account. When you need it for whatever reason you can draw on it with no worries.

When you make regular deposits, you'll reap the benefits and you'll:

Sleep better and relax

Improve your mood

Feel more energetic and productive

Keep up with your kids or grandkids

Clear out the mental cobwebs and focus on tasks

Reduce your level of anxiety and manage stress

Improve your self-esteem and boost my confidence

Lose weight and feel wonderful in the process

Improve your physical appearance

Feel good about myself

Increase your strength and endurance so you can enjoy the activities you love

Enhance sexual desire and performance

Today's Trend of Aging

People today are trying to live longer. They want to be able to do the things they did when they were in their 30's, 40's and 50's. Most people know that they must exercise in order to experience robust health in their advanced years. They want to turn back the clock and be young again. Instead of exercise they try hormone therapy, plastic surgery, crazy diets, etc. They want to look and feel young. Exercise and strength training are one of the best ways to achieve this.

Life expectancy has increased. Most adults are living lifestyles and doing things that weren't imageable thirty years ago. Because of the abundance of information, people have a general idea of what it takes to live healthy. However, most information is for the masses. If you want an extraordinary level of health you must do things that you haven't done or what most people won't do.

Traditional Views on Aging

Aging carries biased and myths that are deeply embedded in society, in particular western society. Traditional western views on aging believe that:

Senility is synonymous with aging.

Older people can't and won't change.

Aging is the same for everyone.

Older people are usually sick.

Older people are supposed to be frail

Older people are supposed to be sedentary sitting in a rocking chair.

It's too late to start a strong and healthy lifestyle.

These false assertions make some older people reluctant to do anything about their health because this is the way they think it should be. Everyone is not the same. Age will take its toll differently on people. Strong and active seniors may become less sick, recover more quickly, and lead fuller lives than others. The rate of decline of fitness is somewhat slower in fit seniors than unfit seniors. Strong and fit seniors remain active and vibrant into their advanced years.

What This Book is About and Who Its For

This book is for those who are over 40 who want to lead strong, full lives into their advanced years with minimal decline in their ability to move and function physically.

Why over 40?

Because according the U.S. Department of Health and Human Service and Harvard University that is the age when people start to lose their muscle mass and muscle tissue.

Why are we concentrating on muscle tissue?

Because losing it can be attributed to many aliments including slower metabolism, loss of energy, Type II diabetes, and osteoporosis. So, in order to slow or reverse muscle loss people must participate in some type of physical activity.

Most exercises and activities will suffice. So, if you enjoy jogging, cycling, swimming, hiking, walking, yoga, Pilates or whatever then do it.

In fact, I encourage it. If you love to train using videos, P90x, Beachbody, Jane Fonda, Richard Simmons or whatever, then do it. However, strength training, exercising using resistance, will provide a quicker path to building much needed muscle.

Strength training has usually been perceived as a young person's game, in particular young man's game. However, this is not true. Any age and gender can participate successfully in strength training.

Also:

> This book is also about understanding, loving, and taking care of yourself.

> This book will show you how to develop a brand-new relationship with yourself.

> This book will give you freedom, freedom to feel and look the way you want.

> This book is not only for sedentary but also for those who what more from their body and those who want to feel their best.

> This book is for beginners to resistance training or strength training. Beginners are those who:

>> Never exercised or trained in their entire life.

>> Haven't exercised since physical education class in school 25, 35, or 50 years ago.

>> Have trained but lack the skills to perform movements correctly.

Have little to no conditioning, meaning they are out of breath after a short walk.

Have little to no strength, mobility, or endurance.

Have the ability to recover from a training session quickly.

If you are intermediate or advance when it comes to resistance training then a lot of information in this book is basic and you heard it at some point. However, there is nothing wrong with reviewing the basics and you might benefit from it.

No one on earth is going to build your body to where you look and feel your best. Only you have the power and control to accomplish it.

It's Never Too Late to Start

This book will start by showing you why you should strength train and the research that says why its beneficial. After that you're going to learn how to train, the anatomy and make up of your muscles, and what it takes to build life extending muscle tissue. You'll learn what equipment to use and some simple exercises to get started.

You'll see how to take care of your strong, growing body through sleep and recovery methods.

Also, in the appendix there is a 7-day food and training log to get you started.

And to keep you on track pick up a copy of *Too Strong to Grow Old 90-Day Training Journal* and use it as a companion to this book.

You'll learn how such a program can be accomplished in three days a week and how you'll experience the following life changing benefits:

Increase your resting metabolic rate to allow you to burn more calories throughout the day.

Increase your stamina and ability to do continuous work

Improve fitness levels, or your body's ability to use oxygen

Perform at higher levels of productivity while becoming less fatigued

Improve your balance and coordination

Increase bone mineral density to prevent osteoporosis

Reduce triglycerides and bad cholesterol

Enhance sexual desire and performance

Increase insulin sensitivity, preventing type 2 diabetes

Improve the function of your immune system

This book is not promising miracles or perfect health and longevity. Building strength is not a guarantee against disease or the perils of life, just as there's no guarantee in investing in the stock market where a crash can ruin the wisest of investors.

However, growing old does not have to guarantee frailty and misery. It's in your power to build and save valuable muscle tissue for when you need it the most, namely in your advanced years. There's no magic or secret to this. And it's available to everyone. If invest the time, effort, desire, and commitment to training your body, will become too strong to grow old.

CHAPTER 1

Benefits of Becoming Strong

Motive, defined as something that prompts a person to act in a certain way or do a certain thing, a reason, an incentive.

Most people know that any type of movement be it physical labor or planned exercise is beneficial for the body. Doctors have always recommended exercise for health going all the way back to the 4th Century BC when Hippocrates said, "walking is man's best medicine."[1]

So, if this assertion is valid then it stands to reason that having a strong body is a motive to improve strength, health, and longevity.

However, some people are not motivated because of this reason. They only start training and exercising after their doctor tells them they will die if they don't. And then some people exercise on their own volition because they realize the benefits of it. They want maximum independence in their advanced years.

So, ask yourself what is your motivation for getting stronger and building muscle. Why put forth the effort, sweating and sacrificing? If you can answer that you will more likely to continue to train long term, as in the rest of your life.

Aging

Why are people trying to stop or reverse aging? Obviously, you can't stop or reverse your chronological age, the number of years you lived on earth. If you're 80 you can't stop yourself from turning 81 or go back to 76. Aging is not considered just in the context of time, as in years, but in the rate at which you let your body decay.

When talking about age we're talking about your biological age rather than your chronological age in years. Your age in years has little to do with how old you are biologically and how old you feel.

We're not talking about cosmetic or visible appearance of age such as receding hairline or sagging skin.

We mean things that are sometimes inevitable due to aging such as decline in hearing, decline in eyesight, slow reaction time etc. However, strength training can help slow aging and many other things.

I'm sure you've ran across people who look 50 at the age of 70. Or others who aged 10 years only in the span of a year. You can say that the latter person has aged or grown old. So, age or being old is relative. You can be 35 and feel old as a result of your life style or you can be active at the age of 75 and feel young and feel great.

The key is to become too strong to grow old, which means building strength and muscle by strength and resistance training so you won't grow old. This will enable you to reverse or slow down the rate of deterioration of your body so you won't end up frail, helpless, and waiting to die.

Not Too Late

Some people treat their bodies like they treat their cars. They drive their bodies for the first 30 years of their lives like they drive a car. They are driving this car, smashing into things, breaking it, not maintaining it, not putting any oil in it. And then by the time they get to 40, 50 or sometimes even 60, they think, "oh crap, I have to actually start maintaining this thing." And by then, they're actually going back and trying to get back to baseline because they haven't even tried to maintain their physical body. Even though for some this may be the case, it's never late and you're never too old to start changing.

For those who are sedentary basically any vigorous aerobic exercise will stave off related muscle decline or Sarcopenia[2,3]. However, if you've been relatively active then your body will need a larger intense stimulus such as strength training[4].

Control

Some people don't treat their bodies as an object of great resource and great value and end up a lot of times playing catch up later in life.

You must recognize that you're in control of your physical body and take full responsibility for its maintenance. You have to figure out for yourself:

> What does it feel like to have healthy bones and healthy teeth?

What does it feel like to have more energy so you can do anything at any time you want?

What is it like when your skin is healthy?

What does it feel like to have optimal blood pressure and digestion system so you can eat what you want?

What does it feel like to have optimal hormone levels?

What does it feel like to have your limbs be limber and be able to move freely without being in pain?

What does it feel like to have your muscles strong and respond to your command so you can engage in your favorite activities?

You have to take account of all of this. It's your responsibility to understand what your body needs to function well and optimally. So, what do you need to be eating? What time do you need to be sleeping? It's your responsibility within this lifetime to develop your body to the maximum of your potential while you are here.

This could involve an athletic pursuit or in something that allows you to tax your body to a peak physical state You will begin to feel not just a physical, but a psychological and physiological change in your state. And the interesting thing about this is a lot of high performers feel like this. That's why some people get a runner's high when they're running, and feel like they could just go for hours.

That's why when you're on a difficult hike, and you get to the top of the peak, the payoff is so great. You climbed a mountain, and your body is tired, but it's not painful. You feel the exertion and the effort, but it's not pain, and your body feels both exhausted and exhilarated. So, this becomes a very rewarding experience, but you have to get to a point where it starts with understanding what is good for your body. You must maintain your health, and understand what your body needs to perform.

Pushing yourself gradually over time takes effort, however when you do, you'll become the master of your body, able to push it past the thing you thought you were previously not capable.

Earlier we talked about your motivation for starting a strength training program. Below are some important reasons and how it will benefit your life.

Slows Aging

Slowing aging is a major reason for starting a strength training program and the main subject of this book. Most people want to slow their aging in some or fashion but don't know how. Strength training will accomplish this.

Strength training slows aging by increasing your Type II muscle fibers, fibers used for intense, heavy, or short duration exercises, which are important in slowing age related muscle decline or Sarcopenia[5,6].

Strength training will greatly slow the aging process, enhancing the quality of your remaining years while maintaining and or increasing your vitality[5].

Helps Your Brain

Let's face it exercise is not easy. You need dedication and commitment to train two to three days a week when it's easy to blow it off and do something else. However, if you can commit to it you can do most things. Strength training gives you the confidence to handle anything mental or physical challenge you face. Exercise can help stimulate parts of your brain that aren't as responsive when you're feeling depressed. It also promotes the release of feel-good brain chemicals. It may also help distract you from your worries and improve your confidence. It releases dopamine that will improve your mood and motivation[7].

Fat loss and Body composition

Most people exercise not only for their health but to look toned, well defined, and fit. Strength training improves your ability to lose body fat improving your body composition[1]. It will increase your lean muscle mass thereby increasing your metabolic rate and burn fat[8].

The more muscle you have the better. It is the key to increasing your resting metabolism or how many calories you burn at rest. This means that the calorie-burning benefits of weights aren't limited to when you are exercising. You may keep burning calories for hours or days afterward[9,10].

Improves Your Sex Life

Strength training improves your ability to have longer, pleasurable, and more intense sex by strengthening the muscles to give you more stamina and optimizes important hormones related to sex drive[11].

A 2008 study conducted at Florida Atlantic University found that men and women who exercised frequently were more likely to rate themselves higher in regards to sexual performance and sexual desirability. However, these researchers found that the improvements in sexual health varied between the two sexes.

Physical activity such as resistance training was shown to prime a woman's body for sexual activity by making her more sensitive to touch and increasing the efficacy of stimuli, while men experience improved sexual function and better orgasms.

Improves Balance

As you get older the loss of muscle mass effects your ability to produce force and stabilize your structure when you are walking or standing. Strength training strengthens your muscles to form a stronger base to keep you stable when you are off balance[12].

A 2013 study published in the Journal of Physical Therapy Science found that after a 12-week randomized controlled trial comparing the effects of strengthening and balance exercises found that after training, the lower limb strength balance of the individuals in the training group had significantly improved older persons[13.]

Improves Mood

Everyone needs some type of mental boost and strength training may be your answer. It can improve your cognitive abilities, self-esteem, and mood.

A 2010 report published in the American Journal of Lifestyle Medicine that resistance training was shown to improve several aspects of cognition in healthy adults. They found that one of the most striking effects of resistance training was the marked improvement in memory and memory-related tasks healthy older adults[14.]

Strength training also improves your mood and gives you the confidence to handle physical and mental situation[14]. Bottom line, when you need a lift, lift weights.

Increases Aerobic Capacity

People perform cardio exercises such as jogging, cycling, and swimming in an effort to improve their heart and increase oxygen capacity. These are all great exercises. however, strength training will do more to increase your aerobic capacity and maximal cardiac output than those exercises[15,16].

Strength training builds muscle mass, thus you will have more muscle cells to consume oxygen. When you breathe deeply during any type of physical exertion your heart beats faster in order to pump as much oxygen to your muscles as possible. Basically, the more muscle you have the greater your use of oxygen[17,18]. The opposite is true, less muscle you have the lower aerobic capacity you have because you have less muscle cell that demand oxygen.

Improves Power

Most tasks or movements you perform throughout your day requires you to overcome inertia, or state or inactivity. Power allows you to overcome this. Power is the rate of speed that allows you to overcome a force.

You can develop the power the necessary to perform tasks efficiently by participating in a strength training program. Power is very important. You may have enough strength to get off the toilet but it will take you all day if you don't have enough power.

Improves Range of Motion

Flexibility is an important component of fitness and in life. It is necessary completing everyday activities with ease. Having the ability to move your joints through a full range of motion without inuring yourself is liberating. You don't need the flexibility of a gymnast. However, you need enough for getting up out of bed, lifting groceries, and vacuuming the floor require a certain level of flexibility.

Flexibility will deteriorate with age if it is not attended to consistently[13,19].

Increases Bone Density

Your muscles are attached to your bones or skeletal system which is a network of levers that enable you to perform various activities. As we age bone mass can decline for several reasons including inactivity and poor nutrition. Bones become prone to fractures even with minor falls. After the age of 40 bone mass declines at a rate of 1% per[21].

Applying stress your bones in the form of strength training can increase bone density and reduce the risk of osteoporosis[20,21].

Improves the Heart

If your heart goes, then you go. Maintaining a healthy heart is not difficult and can be done by anybody at any age. Performing strength training strengthens your heart and lowers the risk of heart disease.

Findings published in *Medicine and Science in Sports Exercise* show that lifting weights for less than an hour per week can reduce the risk of a heart attack or stroke between 40% and 70%. However, the researchers found spending an excessive amount of time in the weight room does not bring additional benefits[22,23].

Also, engaging in strength training lowers your heart rate and dilates your blood vessels increasing blood flow, thereby improving the body's ability to extract oxygen from the[24].

Posture

I'm sure you have seen elderly people with curved upper backs, a pronounced humped posture called Kyphosis. Caused by arthritis, vertebral ligament calcification, and muscle weakness, Kyphosis can affect mobility and locomotion leading to poor use of respiratory muscles.

Your posture will improve by strengthening the upper back muscles and stretching tight chest muscles thereby keeping your back from slouching[25].

Arthritis

Arthritis, which is an inflammation of the joints, come in serval forms. The most common form of arthritis is osteoarthritis. It occurs in older people usually as result of years of wear and tear on the body. It can affect one or multiple joints. According to the Centers for Disease Control over 54 million adults in the United States have arthritis[25].

Carefully selected strength training movements can help people with arthritis by causing the skeletal joints to move which causes the manufacture of synovial fluid. This helps to distribute the fluid over the cartilage, and forces it to circulate throughout the joint space[25].

Back pain

Talk to people you know who are over 40 and most of them will tell you that they have had problems in their lower back at some point in their life. A sedentary lifestyle, which will lead to weak muscles especially those in your core and pelvis, can sometimes lead to back pain or injury.

Strength training helps to strengthen the abdominal muscles, the lower back extensor muscles, the gluteus maximus, gluteus medius, and the hamstring muscles, leading to less pain and dysfunction[26,27]. Modifying daily activities like squatting down to pick up items can also help prevent low back pain or muscle spasms.

Check with your doctor or therapist to determine if your condition is more serious before starting a strength training program and to be sure it's right for your situation.

Knee problems

Whether you're a competitive athlete, a weekend warrior, or a daily walker, dealing with knee pain can put a kink in your favorite activities.

According to the American Academy of Orthopedic Surgeons, you can help reduce the stress on your knee joint by regularly working the muscles around your knee[29,30].

Having stronger muscles can reduce the impact and stress on your knee, and help your joint move more easily. Strength training helps strengthen the structures of the knee, (muscles, tendons, and ligaments) thereby facilitating the ability of the knee to withstand stress[28,29].

CHAPTER 2

Muscle Anatomy

There are many types of muscles located in the human body. However, we're going to concentrate on the skeletal muscles. These muscles are attached to the skeletal system by tough elastic bands of connective tissue called tendons.

The skeletal system, which made up of many types of bones, are used as levers that transmit forces that the muscles generate.

Muscle is made of myofilaments composed of actin and myosin protein strands. These strands slide across each other shortening the muscle to produce movement.

These myofilaments are grouped together to form myofibrils which in turn are bundles in muscle cells. A muscle cell is also called muscle fibers, which are bundled together to form muscle fascicles. These fascicles are bundled to form a complete muscle.

Muscle Fibers

There are several type of muscle fibers. Each has a different job and different characteristics which are detailed below and in Table 1.1.

Type I Muscle Fibers

Type I fibers are small and thin in size and have a high endurance and aerobic capacity. They are low in strength and for the most part weak. They're also referred to as slow twitch fibers because they develop force and relax slowly and have a long twitch time. They are also highly resistance to fatigue. These fibers are good for endurance type exercises that are long in duration such as cycling, distance running, walking, and swimming.

Type II Muscle Fibers

The second type of muscle fibers are called Type II fibers. These come in two varieties. Type IIa and Type IIx. Both types are more alike than they are different. They are both considered fast twitch fibers, which mean they develop force quickly and relax quickly and have a short twitch time. Also, they are both high in strength and power output with Type IIx fibers being the highest. However, they both lack the endurance capacity of the Type I fibers and are larger. Also:

> Type IIa fibers have a high capacity and Type IIx fiber a very high capacity for glycolytic activity, which is the bodies' ability to break down glucose (carbs) to produce energy anaerobically.

> Type IIa fibers are good for short intense activity such as walking up a hill or climbing stairs, tennis, racquetball, and resistance training. See table 1.2.

Type IIx fibers are good for high intense movements and activities such as weightlifting, sprinting, jumping, running from danger. See table 1.2.

Type IIx fibers have very strong fibers and have almost no resistance to fatigue, however they are more susceptible to injury during maximum use[31].

You can't turn Type I fibers into Type II fibers they're set at birth. We can increase the mass and area of muscle by specific training that focuses on that particular muscle fiber type. So, endurance training will increase Type I fibers and power training increases Type II fibers.

Why should you build your muscle?

Simple, to minimize, prevent or even reverse age related muscle decline or atrophy, called Sarcopenia.

Sarcopenia is due to hormonal changes, sedentary lifestyle, reduced protein synthesis and other factors. This muscle fiber atrophy is observed in both Type I and Type II fibers, but more so in Type II[32,33]. Some facts:

Peak levels of muscle mass is reached between the ages of 20 and 40[32]. For people ages 40 to 65 muscle strength declines approximately 20 percent due to aging and disuse[33].

During the fourth decade of life the body loses .5% of muscle mass per year and 1-2% per year after the age of 50 and three percent after age 60[32].

Regular resistance training can lessen muscles loss. However higher training volumes are beneficial to maximize muscle mass as aging progresses[34].

What you should focus on?

If you what to build muscle and build strength you should concentrate on Type II muscle fibers. As you age muscle mass decreases for several reasons. One of those reasons is disuse. When muscle is not used properly it will atrophy or get smaller. This mainly occurs in Type II fibers[31].

As most people age, they become more sedentary. They retire or stop physical activities due to fatigue, sickness, chronic aches and pains or injury. The key is to keep building Type II muscle fiber which responds to training even in advanced age.

The following tables show the characteristics of muscle fiber types and the involvement of muscle fiber types in various activities.

Table 1.1: Characteristics of Muscle Fiber Types

Characteristics	Type I	Type IIa	Type IIx
Power Output	Low	High	High
Endurance	High	Medium	Low
Force Production	Low	Medium	High
Fiber Area	Small	Medium	Large
Resistance to Fatigue	High	Medium	Low
Oxidative Capacity	High	High	Low
Aerobic Enzymes	High	Medium/Low	Low
Anaerobic Enzymes	Low	High	High
Mitochondrial Density	High	High/Medium	Low
Capillary Density	High	Medium	Low

Table 1.2 Involvement of Muscle Fiber Types in Activities

Sport/Activity	Type I	Type IIa, IIx
Basketball	Low	High
Tennis	Low	High
Climbing Stairs	Low	High
Marathon/10K	High	Low
100m Sprint	Low	High
1500m Run	High	Low
Golf	High	Low
Cycling	High	Low
Barbell Squat	High	High
Tai Chi	High	Low
Walking	High	Low
Yoga	High	Low

Phillip J Germany II

CHAPTER 3

Muscle Description

This section will describe the major muscles involved in the exercises and movements that we will deal with. The diagram shows other smaller muscles but we'll only discuss the major ones.

Upper Body

Upper Arm

The Biceps are the muscle of the front upper arm. Its main function is to move the forearm to the shoulder and to rotate the wrist. Example exercises include the biceps dumbbell or barbell curl and the chin-up.

The Triceps, which is located on the back of the arm, consist of three muscles and is a large portion of the upper arm. Its main function is to straighten the arm and bring it down to the body. Example exercises include triceps cable press, triceps dip, and the triceps kickback.

Forearm

The forearm consists of two muscles. The Brachialis and the Brachioradialis. The Brachialis lies deep or underneath the biceps muscle. Its function is to bring the forearm toward the shoulder. The Brachioradialis lies on the outer portion of the forearm and comes into play when the hands are pointing toward your body as you lift your forearm. Example exercise includes the hammer biceps curl.

Shoulder

The Deltoid consist of three muscles and provides mobility to the front, side and back of the shoulder joint. They sit on the joint like a cap. The deltoid's main function is to move the arm away from body. Example exercises include the front arm raise, overhead press, and the lateral arm raise.

Back

The Latissimus Dorsi or Lats are on both sides of the back from the lower portion of the shoulder down to the lumbar region of the back. Its main function is to pull the arm down from overhead and lift the body up toward the shoulders. Exercises include the lat pull-down and the row, either with dumbbells, barbell, bands, rowing machine or rowing a boat.

The Trapezius or traps is a long diamond shaped muscle that runs down the upper part of spine from the base of the skull to the middle of the back. Its main function is to bring the shoulder blades together, shrug the shoulders up and down, and stabilize the shoulder joint when the deltoid muscles moves. Example exercises include the seated row and the shoulder shrug.

Chest

The Pectorals Major covers all of the upper chest. Its main function is to bring the arm across the chest and to move it forward in the shoulder socket. Example exercises include the bench press with a barbell, dumbbell, or bands, and the push-up.

Lower Body

Calves

The calves consist of the Gastrocnemius and the Soleus. The Soleus lies deep beneath the Gastrocnemius Both runs on from behind the knee and attaches to the heel with the Achilles tendon. The main function of both muscles is to raise the heel from the ground standing on your balls of your feet.

Buttocks

Gluteus Maximus or the muscles of the buttocks run from the rear portion of the pelvis to the upper leg. Its main function is to extend the hip. An example exercise includes the prone straight leg lift.

Upper Leg

The Quadriceps consist of four muscles on the front thigh, the rectus femoris, vastus intermedius, lateralis, and medialis. Its function is to extend the knee joint. A common exercise includes the seated knee extension or stepping up.

The Hamstrings consists of several muscles on the back of the thigh, the Biceps Femoris, Semitendinosus, and the Semimembranosus. Their main function is to bring the heel to toward the back and move the leg backward. Example exercises include the lying, seated or standing leg curl, the bridge, and the stiff leg deadlift.

The Mid-Section and Abdominals

The Rectus Abdominus lie on the front of the mid-section. It is sometimes referred to as the six a pack. Its function is to bring the rib cage toward the pelvis. The muscle fibers run vertically on the mid-section and lies near the surface. Common exercises are the crunch or sit-up.

The Obliques are located on the sides of the mid-section near the waist. Its function is to stabilize and rotate the torso. Example exercises includes a crunch with rotation or the truck twist.

The Transversus abdominis runs horizontally deep across the lower mid-section. It stabilizes the lumbar area of the spine and compresses the contents of the abdomen. Drawing in the stomach or pulling the navel in toward the spine like a vacuum or sucking in your gut are common movement.

MAJOR MUSCLE GROUPS	INDIVIDUAL MUSCLES
Quadriceps (Front leg muscles)	Rectus femoris, Vastus lateralis, Vastus medialis.
Hamstrings (Back leg muscles)	Semitendinosus, Semimembranosus, Biceps femoris.
Chest	Pectoralis major, Pectoralis minor.
Back	Teres major, Latissimus dorsi, Trapezius, Erector spinae, Rhomboids.
Shoulders	Anterior deltoid, Medial deltoid, Posterior deltoid
Abdominals	Rectus Abdominis, Obliques
Calves	Gastrocnemius, Soleus.
Glutes	Gluteus maximus, Glutes minimus.
Biceps	Biceps brachii, Brachialis.
Triceps	Triceps brachii

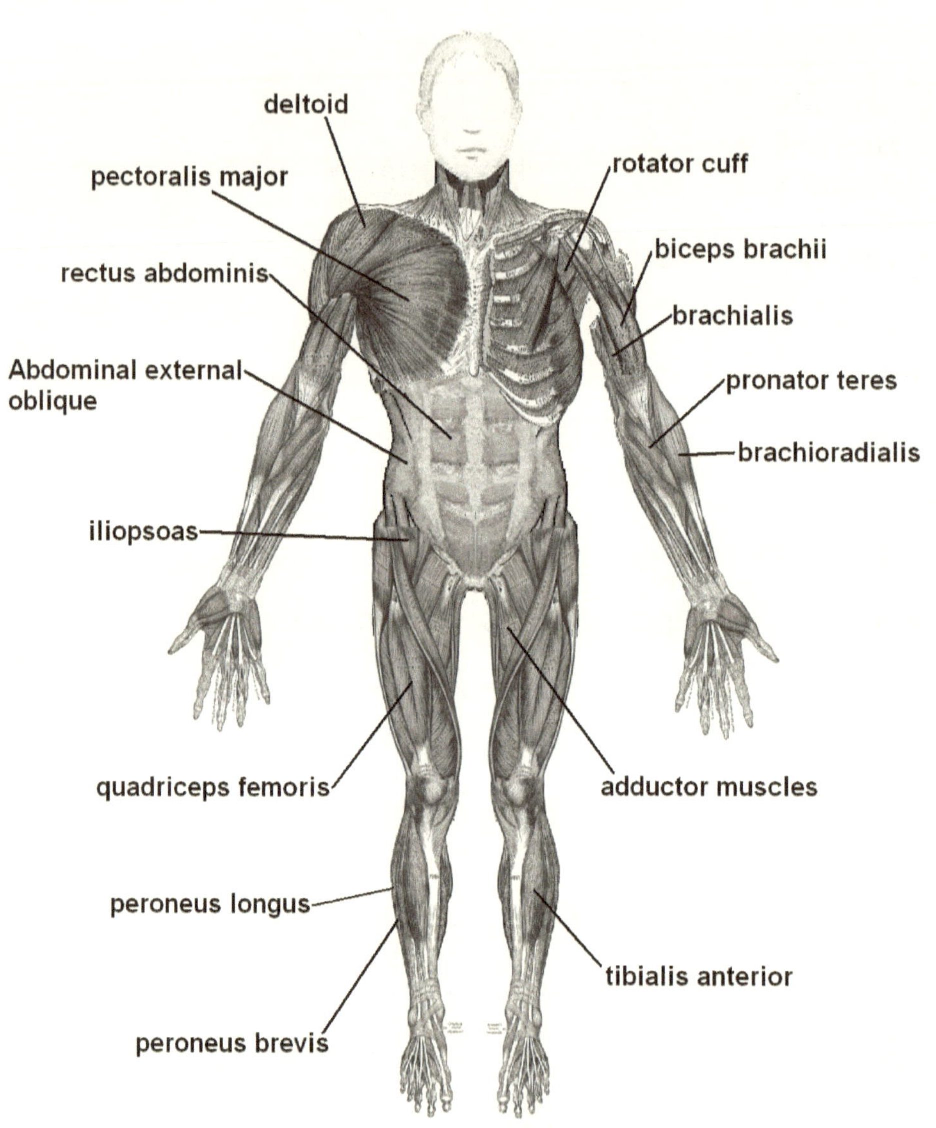

deltoid
pectoralis major
rectus abdominis
Abdominal external oblique
iliopsoas
quadriceps femoris
peroneus longus
peroneus brevis
rotator cuff
biceps brachii
brachialis
pronator teres
brachioradialis
adductor muscles
tibialis anterior

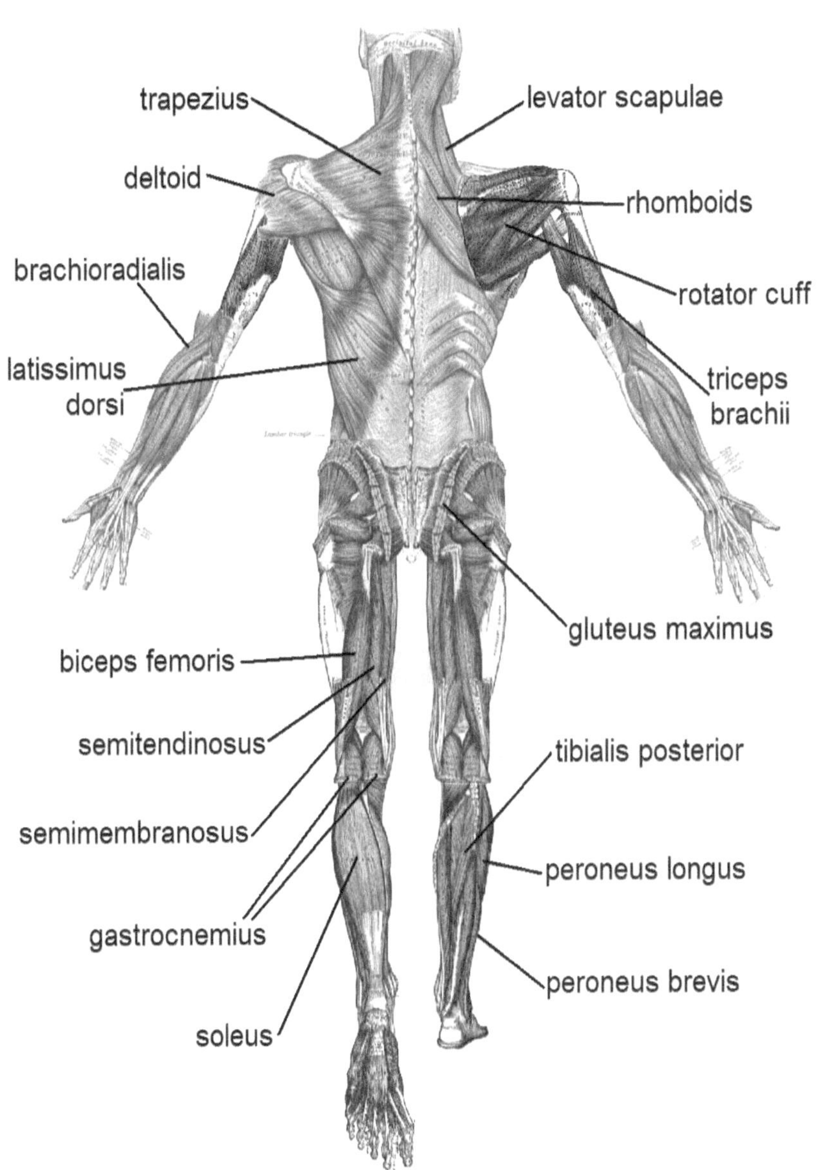
trapezius
levator scapulae
deltoid
rhomboids
brachioradialis
rotator cuff
latissimus
dorsi
triceps
brachii
gluteus maximus
biceps femoris
semitendinosus
tibialis posterior
semimembranosus
peroneus longus
gastrocnemius
peroneus brevis
soleus

Muscle Group	Multi-joint (Compound) Movement	Single-joint (Isolation) Movement
Chest	Push-ups, Presses, Dips	Cable crossovers, Dumbbell Fly
Shoulders	Presses, Upright rows	Side Raises
Back	Rows, Pull-ups, Pull-downs	Pullovers
Quadriceps (Front leg muscles)	Squats, Leg press, Lunges	Leg extensions
Hamstrings (Back leg muscles)	Stiff-legged deadlifts, Squats	Leg curls, Back extension
Glutes	Squats, Good mornings, Kickbacks	Hip extension, Lateral leg raise

CHAPTER 4

Building Muscle

Whenever you see a home or skyscraper, it didn't just come up out of the ground. An architect and developer created a picture their mind as to how the structure should look and function. However, in order to see the fulfilment of his vision, when designing and building that structure, the architect must adhere to certain laws and principles of physical science in order to get the best out of the materials that are used.

Likewise, you should have a vision of how you want your body to look and perform in order to get the best from it. In order to achieve that goal that you must adhere to certain principles, principles that you can control which will yield a high-performance body that will last a long time.

So, the goal here is to build and develop strength by building muscle and stop or reverse age-related muscle decline and all the things that go with it. Accomplishing this is not easy. The following are some principles that you'll need to know in order to successfully build strength.

Anabolism and Catabolism

Your body operates and functions through a number of biochemical reactions and processes that's involved with your body's metabolism. Anabolism and catabolism of molecules are the two major reactions involved building of your body. Both are occurring constantly and simultaneously.

When anabolism is greater than catabolism, growth occurs. When catabolism is greater than anabolism the loss of tissues or non-growth occurs.

This building up and breaking down of molecules come from the foods we consume consisting of protein, carbohydrates, and fats in the form of amino acids, glucose, fatty acids, ketones, and lactic acid.

The following factors have an effect on anabolism and catabolism:

When you eat.

What you eat.

When you train.

Type of training.

Your Hormones.

Your Stress Levels.

Tension

Tension is generated in the muscle to overcome the resistance that is being lifted. This can also be described as stress on the muscle or force generated in the muscle.

Time Under Tension

The more time it takes for your muscle to work is called time under tension. This causes more chemical build up in the muscle which leads to increased protein synthesis and stronger muscles.

Progressive Overload

Progressive overload is simply doing slightly more than the previous training session. You can accomplish this by increasing the amount of weight lifted, completing more repetitions, which is one complete movement of an exercise, or by completing sets, which are several repetitions. This applies to all exercises. For example, if you run, run slightly longer than the previous run.

Muscle damage

This does not refer to pain or an injury. Muscle damage in this context refers to the localized muscle tissue damage in the form of micro tears to the contractile proteins and surface membrane of the working or worked muscle. As a result, your muscles become sore. This soreness is called Delayed Onset Muscle Soreness or DOMS. This is the soreness you experience in a muscle 18-48 hours after training hard. Your muscles will adapt and respond by building new tissue.

Metabolic Stress.

This is the chemical reaction of lactate, hydrogen ion, and phosphate inside muscle cells. This process stimulates protein synthesis which is needed to build muscle, at the same time decreasing the possibility of muscle breakdown.

Methods to control your strength building

Using the principles above along with the following methods you can control and manipulate your strength building program to achieve your goals.

Intensity

This is the amount of weight you lift or how hard you work. For example, doing 30 push-ups may be difficult, but is considered low intensity compared to doing 5 push-ups with someone on your back, which is considered high intensity.

Also, if you train with a certain amount of weight, you would use a percentage of your one rep max (RM). Your one rep max is the heaviest amount of weight you can lift for one time only.

For example, if you were tested and found that your one rep max is 100 pounds then the weight you use too train with would be a percentage of that. The percentage depends on your goals for training. If you want to get strong you would lift a higher percentage. If you were training for endurance you would choose a lower percentage.

Volume

Volume is the number of exercises you do over a particular time period. For example, let's say you currently train three per days a week. If you increased it to five days per week then you would be increasing the number of exercises you do over that period thereby increasing your volume.

Another way to increase your volume would be to do more exercise at each workout. For example, if you complete six exercises of various types in a 45-minute workout in order to increase the volume you would do seven exercises in that time period. Conversely if you wanted to decrease the volume and do less you would just decrease the number of exercises or days per week you train.

When it comes to designing your training program volume and intensity are inversely related. If you work at higher intensities you should work at lower volume. If you work at lower intensities you would work at a higher volume.

For example, if you perform a movement that is 90 percent of your one rep maximum (1RM) that's considered high intensity. If you perform a movement that is 75-85 percent of your 1RM that is medium intensity and 60-75 percent of your 1RM is low intensity. Medium and high intensity is the levels where you build strength and muscle mass.

Rest intervals. Rest between sets

Rest intervals are the amount of time from the last repetition of a set to first repetition of the next set. The duration of your rest between sets is crucial to your training and strength development. As we saw earlier the harder your muscle works the more tension is developed. For building strength, you would rest longer between sets. For muscles growth and endurance, you would decrease your rest time.

Resting between sets is a necessary and an important part of training. It allows your muscles and nervous system to recover so you will be able to perform the next set. The following are some more considerations for rest intervals:

You need more rest between sets if you are performing a high intense set.

You need more rest between sets if you are performing difficult exercises such as the squat or pull-ups.

You need more rest between sets if you are performing multi-joint exercises such as the squat or push-ups.

If you are lifting heavy weight or training for maximum strength your rest period between sets should be in the 3-5-minute range.

Compared with a person training for endurance, fat loss, or larger muscles (hypertrophy) they would rest for 30 seconds to 2 minutes.

When training with heavy weight you should rest until you are completely recovered from the last set regardless of time.

Keep in mind that when you're training for strength you should not perform other exercises or some type of cardio between sets to keep your heart rate up. That's interval training, and there is a time and place for that. However, the focus here is building strength and increasing muscle mass for overall body improvement, health, and avoiding age related muscle decline.

Frequency and Number of Training Days Per Week

Frequency is related to volume, in that the number of exercise sessions in a given time period affects your ability to train and affects your results. The amount of time allowed between workout sessions is important because depending on the intensity of your workout you would need the appropriate amount of time off until your next workout.

For example, if you went all out in a workout at a high intensity you would need more time off until your next workout of the week thereby decreasing the number of days or frequency you'd train in that week. This time period between workouts is referred to as recovery time which we'll discuss later.

Finding time to train is challenging. Life can and will get in the way. Responsibilities such as bills, family, work, the house, the car, taxes, the holidays, children, etc. Add that to the stress of training and it will have a tremendous effect on your body and you'll risk overtraining.

For the beginner starting out or the person that hasn't exercised in a long-time training three to five days a week is a good starting point and probably will be more effective. However, unless you're a serious amateur or professional athlete training six or seven days a week is not advisable[35]. More is not better. There is the law of diminishing returns. Your body, mind, and nervous system can only handle so much.

Take the following factors into account when planning your training and deciding how many days a week to train.

Your Goals

Your health and fitness goals will determine the number of days you will train. One of your major goals as you age should include increasing your strength. To accomplish this, you should train at a medium to high intensity. Careful planning is important. Overtraining is more detrimental than undertraining.

Your Age

The number of days you train will depend on your age. A person who is 30 usually can train more days a week than a person who is 65 or 70. One of the main reasons is recovery time between workouts. As we age, we need more time for our muscles, joints, tendons, and central nervous system to recover from the previous workout[36].

Is this ALWAYS the case, no. There will be some 65-year-olds that can train hard multiple days in a row, but those are exceptions[37].

Your Job

If you're an accountant, an administrative assistant, a bus driver or any other job that requires you to sit more than you stand or walk you'll be able to handle more weekly workouts than if you're working 12 hours in a steel plant or digging ditches.

Your Family

If you have a busy family life with small or teen-age children or if you're taking care of elderly family members this will be a factor in your weekly training frequency because this extra responsibility and stress will take its toll on your body.

Stress

Chronic everyday stress is taken into account when deciding how many days a week to workout. Hard training is a stress on your body and nervous system. Add to that major stressors such as job deadlines, bills, relationships, deaths and other stress producing events can take its toll. However, it's the cumulative effect of small nettlesome stressors such as traffic, long lines at the store, constant interruptions can have an even bigger effect on your life and training[38.]

Recovery

How you recover is probably the biggest factor. Recovery is needed to rest your muscles, nervous system, and your joints. We'll discuss this in more detail later.

Exercise selection

Exercise selection is an important factor in becoming stronger. For the most part a great majority of resistance movements will do the job if the above principles are adhered to.

However, some movements lend themselves to causing better overall strength and development, getting more bank for your buck so to speak. For example, if you're pressed for time and trying to get a good workout in, doing one arm bicep curls is not as efficient as doing bench presses.

If done right both exercises will increase strength only that the bicep curl is working basically one muscle while the bench press is working several muscles.

CHAPTER 5

Getting Started

The previous chapter we talked about the principles and methods of building strength. However how do you accomplish this and what should you use?

As mentioned in chapter 4 in order to build a home or skyscraper an architecture needs certain tools to create plans for the project and the construction worker need tools and equipment to erect the structure. They need to use those tools in the proper fashion in order to achieve the desired results.

Your body is no different. You as the architect of building your strength must use the proper tools and equipment in the proper way in order to achieve the desired results. This chapter will discuss the tools, equipment, and methods you can use to build your strength.

Safety First

Exercise of all forms is exciting, exhilarating, and good for you. However, when it comes to strength training safety is important and should be observed. Before jumping into an exercise or training program of any kind you should take several precautions.

Medical Clearance

Medical clearance should be obtained before starting a training program. A pre-existing health issue could affect your ability to train and hinder any progress. This is especially important for those over the age of 40. Your doctor will tell you if certain movements or exercises are off limits. You should do this whether you train by yourself, at home, in a gym, fitness center, or anywhere.

If you work with a personal fitness trainer, they will definitely require a medical clearance, if they don't, find another trainer. With the amount of effort and intensity you'll put into training a medical clearance can benefit your long-term well-being.

Hydrate

Adequate fluids are a must if you plan to train hard. Thirst is not an indicator that your body need fluids. If you wait until your thirsty, dehydration may have started. You should hydrate before, during, and after training, preferably with water. You can drink sports drinks, however just know that they are composed of simple carbohydrates and they are calorically dense.

Lifting Belt

When you are lifting heavy weight during strength training some movements will involve your lower back. Wearing a lift belt will help to protect it from undue stress. Be advised, a belt will not PREVENT a low back injury. It will only alleviate the stress applied to the lumbar region. You should wear a belt primarily for heavy squats and deadlifts when lifting very heavy weight such as 80% of your one rep max or higher.

Warm up and Stretching

Warm up

For whatever reason there are some people who overlook and ignore warming up before a workout. This is a serious mistake. The warm-up is necessary for anyone of any age who trains and especially people over the age of 40. The following are some key points for a warm-up:

It prepares the body for movements that it may not be used to or that you do not do often.

The warm-up gets the proper blood flow to your muscles.

The warm-up prepares your muscles for work at a high level.

The warm-up should be simple and not too taxing. You don't want to get too tired before your workout.

It improves your ability to recover and possibly lessen the chance for serious injury.

The warm-up can be split into two types, general and specific. You should always perform the general warm-up first. It should consist of movements that increase the temperature of your body and increase blood circulation. Your muscles will produce more force which will lead to more weight lifted or more reps, a better workout, and better results.

General Warm-up

A general warm-up can consist of any light cardiovascular exercise, jogging, cycling, rowing, yoga or even walking and swinging your arms. Basically, any movement you enjoy that will get your body warm and break a light sweat. However, it should be performed at a low intensity and should not lead to fatigue. After you perform a general warm up you can proceed to the second type which is the specific warm-up.

Specific Warm-up

The specific warm-up targets the particular muscle or muscle group that you will train during your workout.

A specific warm-up takes muscles through their full range of motion. You use movements that are similar to the actual activity in your workout. The specific warm-up should be the same or as close to the actual training movement as possible. For example, if you are going to train your legs you would perform a couple of light sets body weight squats as a specific warm-up.

The amount of time you spend warming up depends on several factors. For example, a longer warm up would be in order if you are training first thing in the morning or if you are training in colder weather. There are no rules as far as the length of time. You should warm up to a point to where you feel comfortable and that your body is ready for major activity.

Stretching

Everyone needs some degree of flexibility. However, most people don't need the flexibility of a yogi or and gymnast. You just need enough to meet to the demands of your activity.

Flexibility refers to the ability of your joints to move through their full range of motion. In order for this to occur your muscles must be supple and elongated enough, and stretching will accomplish this.

Stretching is important to help prepare the muscles for activity and achieve a desired level of flexibility. Some key points concerning stretching include:

When stretching, go only as far as when you feel a slight tension in the muscle.

Stretch slowly and not too far.

If you stretch too far your body employs a stretch reflex causing the muscle to contract which is not the desired effect you are looking for before a hard workout.

The stretch reflex is a neural impulse the body sends when a muscle is stretched too far.

You should stretch the entire body regardless if you're training the upper body or lower body.

Stretching before exercise does not prevent injury[39]. However chronically short and tight muscles can be a precursor to an injury.

Stretching doesn't prevent muscle soreness which is sometimes experienced after an intense workout[39, 40].

There are two main ways of stretching, static and dynamic. There are a few other types but they fall under the heading of one of these two.

Static

Static stretching is the most common form of stretching. People usually do it before a workout. However, doing it before strength training can be counterproductive as it can temporarily lower your strength levels[41].

Static stretching is beneficial after training for recovery and increasing mobility. When performing a static stretch move slowly into the desired position and hold the stretch for 20-60 seconds. Never jerk or bounce.

Dynamic

Dynamic stretching involves active movements that stretch the muscles but not held in position. It resembles a specific movement or motion related to an exercise or a sports movement. Dynamic stretching is used by those to increase range of motion for sports skills.

Swinging your arms through a full range of motion is an example of dynamic stretching. This is the type of stretching you should do before strength training[42]. An example of a dynamic stretching routine would be swinging your arms for a particular number of reps or for time like 30 seconds. Other movements could include leg swings or kicks, air punches, squatting etc.

Remember to warm-up before any stretching, dynamic or static, and never stretch a cold muscle. Be advised that achieving a good range of motion is important however excessive flexibility can be detrimental as is can lead to a decrease in joint stability.

Exercises

Compound and Isolation Movements

Compound

Compound exercises, also called multi-joint movements, involve exercising muscles using more than one joint. For example, the squat is a compound exercise because it involves movement of the hip joint, the knees, and to a lesser degree the ankles. It also involves major muscles such as the quadriceps, hamstrings, hip flexors, and glutes.

When building strength, which is our major focus, its best to perform compound movements. You get more bang for your buck because you're working multiple muscles in one exercise which will cause better overall development in those muscles[43].

Also, with compound movements:

You'll tend to lose more fat and improve your overall fitness.

You can use heavier weights, which is important if your goal is to increase your strength. However, compound exercises are taxing, so you should be careful with the amount of weight you use.

Multiple joints share in the work load.

Planning is critical. Because of the many muscles involved, overtraining can occur and could affect subsequent training sessions.

Correct form is very important for this type of training.

You'll strengthen not only your muscles but also your connective tissues that support those muscles. This is important because if your connective tissues are not supportive enough you will be prone to injury.

Develops a solid strength foundation, especially if you're a beginner.

Isolation

Isolation exercises involves exercising your muscles using only one joint. For example, when you perform the bicep curl you only move one joint, your elbow, when contracting your bicep and lifting the weight.

This type of training is use by those want to target certain muscles, for example a bodybuilder or fitness model who want to develop more defined biceps.

Also, isolation exercises:

Uses fewer muscle groups at one time requiring less intensity and energy than compound exercises.

Allows you to use lighter weight.

Targets a particular muscle.

Equipment

When it comes to building a strong body your choices for equipment are many. You can start getting stronger, looking good, and feeling great with minimal to no equipment at all. You can start your program with equipment that fits your lifestyle and budget. Choose equipment that you like, that's not complicated to use, and that will challenge your body. Here are some examples.

Barbells

A barbell set is a great way to build lasting strength and overall fitness. Barbells are probably the most efficient at using your muscles and less time consuming. Most if not all barbell movements are compound movements so this forces you to use more muscles and more effort in an exercise, allowing greater strength and power to be achieved.

Barbell sets are usually sold as a 300-pound set. This consist of a seven foot, 45-pound bar, two 45, 35, 25, and 10-pound plates along with four five-pound plates and two, 2.5 bar collars which go on either end of the bar to keep the plates form sliding off.

Also:

> Barbell training develops stabilizer muscles, the smaller muscles that supports a body part to allow larger muscles to contract.

> Barbells are more versatile than machines and less expensive.

> Barbell training matches patterns of your normal movement from a biomechanical perspective.

However, there are some drawbacks to using barbells. They can become time consuming when changing weights and plates. Also, with barbells you need more space for storage and usage, and it can be expensive to obtain a good barbell set.

Dumbbells

Training with dumbbells is similar to training with barbells in that they allow stabilizer muscles to come into play in most if not all movements. Dumbbells are versatile and simple to use.

There are several types of dumbbells that are more common in todays' training.

> **Solid dumbbells.** These dumbbells come with spherical, cylindrical and octagonal ends.

> **Power Block.** These dumbbells are adjustable up to approximately 50-55 pounds in 2.5 increments. They

come as a square block or octagonal. They take up less space and cheaper than a full set.

Various others. Other dumbbell types include fixed plate and Olympic.

Some drawbacks with dumbbells are that you need lots of dumbbells of various weights as you progress in strength because the lighter dumbbells will become easy over time. Also buying many dumbbells can be expensive and you'll need lots of storage space.

Kettlebells

Kettlebells have become a part of modern fitness as much as any other piece of equipment. These ominous looking devices have been around for decades in the Soviet Union and in a scant number of gyms in the United States. However, they made a comeback in the U.S. around the late 90's.

Kettlebells are everywhere and everybody are espousing the benefits of them, Also:

Popular movements such like the swing, get-up, and squat can build core stability, endurance, power, strength, and overall fitness.

The drawback is that they are expensive and they come in unusual increments (16, 24, and 32 kilos or 35,53, and, 70 pounds).

However, if one kettlebell becomes easy then you have to buy another one in order to continue building strength progressively.

Bands

These include large rubber bands or surgical tubing with handles on the ends. The degree of elasticity is the source of these band's resistance. These devices come in various thicknesses so if a person wants more resistance, they would choose the corresponding band.

The advantage is that they are inexpensive, simple to use, and convenient. However, the drawbacks are that you're limited in progression of resistance and they could wear out and break after prolonged use.

Machines

Enter into the majority of commercial gyms and you'll find various machines that can work all of your muscles. There are machines that will train the chest, arms, legs, abdominals, the back, neck, obliques, shoulders, and calves.

Most machines are straightforward and simple to use. However, there are times when you'll need the help of gym personnel or your personal trainer to use one. Machines also have placards posted on them that display the instructions on how to properly use the machine and the muscle groups that are worked.

One great advantage of using machines is that they are easy to use and they allow for faster workout because you don't have to change plates or walk and grab dumbbells

A major disadvantage of machines is that the movement you perform in most machines are not natural movements. Because these machines are made for people of average height, weight, and build, you are forced to move along a movement pattern is predetermined. Another disadvantage is that most machines isolate a muscle, so the surrounding supporting muscles or stabilizer muscles surrounding it are not worked, which is not how natural movement pattern is designed.

Calisthenics and Bodyweight, Including Wrist and Ankle Weights

Using your bodyweight as the main source of resistance is a great way for a beginner to start a strength training program.

Bodyweight training includes push-ups, pull-ups, chin-ups, jumping jacks, trampolines, and much more. Even running, speed walking, and jogging can be classified as calisthenics and bodyweight movements because you are using your own weight in the movement.

Remember that in order to make progress and gain strength your muscles must receive more stress each time you train, progressive overload of your muscles.

Also, some calisthenics are designed to improve endurance or flexibility so choose wisely which movements you would use to improve strength and build muscle mass.

As you progress in your training performing calisthenics and bodyweight movements will become less demanding as your body will adapt to the stress that is placed on it, namely your bodyweight. In order to progressively overload your muscles, you can wear ankle and wrist weights or even use small light dumbbells during the movements.

Basic Exercises

There are thousands of exercises that exist for every part of the body which makes training exciting. However, we're going to focus on compound movements using barbells, dumbbells, and bodyweight. Also, you can use kettlebells, canned foods, jugs of water, and bottles of water as substitutes for dumbbells.

However, before you perform any exercise you must learn to perform it correctly. This means learning the proper form and becoming skilled at a particular exercise using little to no weight. Doing so will allow your body to get used to the correct mechanics and prevent injury.

Also, with compound movements, there will be crossover of muscles used, so take that into consideration when designing your program and planning your recovery.

Arms

Barbell Curls

Stand with your feet shoulder width apart, keeping your knees slightly bent.

Hold the barbell with a shoulder width underhand grip with your arms down to your thighs.

Slowly raise the bar towards your upper chest, squeezing your muscles and isolating the biceps.

Hold this position for 1 count and then return back to the starting position.

Do not:

> Use momentum to lift the weight.
>
> Lean back excessively

Dumbbell Curls

> Stand with your feet shoulder width apart, keeping your knees slightly bent.

Hold each dumbbell with a shoulder width underhand grip with your arms down to your thighs.

Slowly raise both dumbbells towards your upper chest, squeezing your muscles and isolating the biceps.

Hold this position for 1 count and then return back to the starting position.

Note:

Do not use momentum to lift the weight or lean back excessively.

Triceps Kickbacks

Stand with your knees slightly flexed, bending forward at the waist.

Keep your upper back straight.

Hold the dumbbell with your elbow bent at a 90-degree angle at your side.

Straighten your arm at the elbow.

Only bend your elbow and do not raise your shoulder.

Return to the starting position.

Band curls

Place a band under your feet and hold the handles palms forward in your hands.

Stand with your feet shoulder width apart, knees slightly bent.

Curl your arms up.

Return to the starting position.

Shoulders

Barbell Overhead Press

Stand with your feet shoulder width apart keeping your back straight and chest up.

Pick the barbell the floor and raise it to shoulder level. Your palms should face away from you.

Press the barbell straight up until your arms are straight.

Lower the barbell back to shoulder level and repeat.

After you complete all of your repetitions place the barbell on the floor.

Dumbbell Overhead Press

Stand with your feet shoulder width apart keeping your back straight and chest up.

Pick the dumbbells off the floor and raise them to shoulder level with your palms facing away from you.

Press the both dumbbells straight up until your arms are straight. As an alternative you can raise the dumbbells by alternating each arm.

Lower the dumbbells back to shoulder level and repeat.

After you complete all of your repetitions place the dumbbells on the floor.

Lateral Raises

Stand up straight with your feet shoulder width apart holding a dumbbell in each hand down by your sides with your palms facing downward and arms straight out.

Raise your arms to shoulder level.

Return back to the starting position.

Band Lateral Raise

Stand on a band so that it is evenly distributed to be pulled by each arm. You may need two bands, one for each arm.

Grab the handles keeping your arms down and rested at your side.

Use your shoulders to raise your hands above your sides so that they are at shoulder level then lower the handles back down to the starting position.

Band Press

Begin by standing on a band so that it is evenly distributed to be pulled by each arm. You may need two bands, one for each arm.

Hold the handles and bring your arms up to shoulder level.

Use your shoulders, and raise your hands over head.

Lower the handles back down to the starting position.

Chest

Band Bench Press

Start with placing a band under the leg of the bench where your head will be resting or you can use a shorter band and place it under your upper back.

If you don't have access to a bench, lay on the floor and place a shorter band under your upper back.

Lay flat down on a flat bench or floor, grab the handle of the band, one in each hand at shoulder width.

Push your arms up toward the sky until your arms are straight.

Return back to the starting position.

Barbell Bench Press

Lie with your back flat on a bench with your feet firmly on the ground and the bar resting on the bench's rack.

Slowly lift the bar off the rack and hold it above your chest, this is the starting position.

Lower the bar down until it slightly touch against your chest.

Hold this position briefly and make sure you have complete control of the bar.

Raise the bar back up to the starting position.

Place the bar on the rack after you complete your set.

Dumbbell Bench Press

Start by picking the dumbbells that you can manage, holding them at your sides and then sitting on the edge of a flat bench.

Using your thighs and thrusting of your arms to lift the weights onto your legs in your starting position.

Lean back onto the bench and on the motion down, push the dumbbells up about an inch high above your chest as this is your starting position.

The dumbbells should be aligned with the middle of your chest and then slowly push the dumbbells up above your body using mostly your chest and triceps for the motion upward.

Stop the motion of the exercise as soon as your arms are straight and the dumbbells are directly above your chest.

Hold for 1 count, then return back to the starting position.

On the return motion down, do not let gravity do the work or drop the dumbbells, you should be resisting gravity of the way down.

Push-up

Start by kneeling on the floor or on a mat.

Place your arms shoulder width apart on the mat.

Lift your knees off the ground and extend your legs, keep your head and neck in line with your body.

Spread your feet slightly apart. Only your hands and toes should be touching the floor.

Inhale as you lower yourself down towards the ground until your chest almost touches the ground.

Hold for 1 count at the bottom position and then while exhaling return back up to the starting position.

If you are unable to perform a standard push-up try the easier variations below until you progress to the standard push-up.

Push-up, on Knees

Start by kneeling on the floor or on a mat.

Place your arms shoulder width apart on the mat. Your torso should be at an angle, keep your head and neck in line with your body.

Inhale as you lower yourself down towards the ground until your chest almost touches the ground.

Hold for 1 count at the bottom position and then while exhaling return back up to the starting position.

Wall Push-up

Place your arms shoulder width apart on a wall.

Move your feet back so you are leaning against the wall. Your torso should be at a slight angle.

Spread your feet slightly apart.

Inhale as you lower yourself down towards the wall until your chest almost touches it.

Hold for 1 count at the bottom position and then while exhaling return back to the starting position.

Torso Elevated Push-up

Place your arms shoulder width apart on a table, bench or stable surface that is high than your knees.

Move your feet back so you are leaning against the surface. Your body should be at a slight angle.

Spread your feet slightly apart.

Inhale as you lower yourself down towards the surface until your chest almost touches it.

Hold for 1 count at the bottom position and then while exhaling return back up to the starting position.

Band Chest Fly

Start with placing a band under the leg of the bench where your head will be resting or you can use a shorter band and place it under your upper back.

If you don't have access to a bench lay on the floor and place a shorter band under your upper back.

Hold the band handle in each hand keeping your elbows slightly bent and arms out at your sides facing straight down towards the ground so that you feel a stretch in your chest.

Bring your hands together above your chest, as if you're hugging someone. hold this position for 1 count.

Return to the starting position and repeat.

Dumbbell Fly

Lie on a bench or the floor

Hold a dumbbell in each hand keeping your elbows slightly bent and arms out at your sides facing straight down towards the ground so that you feel a stretch in your chest.

Bring your hands together above your chest, as if you're hugging someone. Hold this position for 1 count.

Return the dumbbells back to their starting position and repeat for as many reps and sets as desired.

Back

Pull ups/Chin ups

Find a bar high enough that you can reach on your tip toes or lower.

Start by grabbing the crossbar with an overhand grip, letting your body hang from the bar and keeping your arms straight, this your starting position.

Once in position, slowly pull yourself up so that your chin is higher than the bar, squeezing your back muscles and lats and hold for 1 count.

Return back to the starting position.

Variation: to make this easier you can place one foot on the ground or a chair and perform the pull up.

Underhand Grip Pull ups/Chin ups

Find a bar high enough that you can reach on your tip toes or lower.

Start by grabbing the crossbar with an underhanded grip, letting your body hang from the bar and keeping your arms straight, this your starting position.

Once in position, slowly pull yourself up so that your chin is higher than the bar, squeezing your back muscles and lats and hold for 1 count.

Return back to the starting position.

Variation: You can place one foot on the ground and perform the pull up.

Neutral Grip Pull ups/Chin ups

Find a set of parallel bars, rings, or handles to where your palms are facing inward.

Make sure the bars are high enough that you can reach on your tip toes or lower.

Start by grabbing the bars with a neutral grip, palms facing in, letting your body hang from the bar and keeping your arms straight, this your starting position.

Once in position, slowly pull yourself up so that your chin is higher than the bar, squeezing your back muscles and lats and hold for 1 count.

Return back to the starting position.

Variation: You can place one foot on the ground and perform the pull up.

Note: Your choice of grip will depend on your shoulder or elbow health. Choose what's comfortable. If nothing is comfortable, choose an alternative back exercise.

Barbell Rows

Stand in front of a barbell with your feet shoulder width apart.

Grab the bar with a shoulder width grip, underhand or overhand, then lift the bar up off of the ground until your back is at an angle, this is the starting position.

Keep your head up and your back straight. Do not round your back.

Raise the bar up towards your upper abdominals using a controlled motion and continue until the bar is almost touching your body. Do not jerk the bar up.

Hold for 1 count, squeezing your back muscles and then lower the bar back to the starting position.

Dumbbell Rows

Stand with your feet shoulder width apart and hold a dumbbell in each hand.

Bend over until your back is at an angle, this is the starting position. Keep your head up and your back straight. Do not round your back.

Raise the dumbbells up on your sides towards your chest using a controlled motion and continue until the dumbbells are almost touching your lower chest. Do not jerk the dumbbells up.

Hold for 1 count, squeezing your back muscles and then lower the dumbbells back to the starting position.

One Arm Row

Start by kneeling over the side of a bench by placing the knee and hand of the supporting arm on the bench and then position the opposite foot on the floor.

If you don't have a bench you can just place your hand on a table, chair or some other sturdy support. Or you can just bend at the waist with your back strait and at a slight angle.

Grab a dumbbell from the floor opposite of the side supporting the body and pull the dumbbell up slowly on your sides to your chest, feeling a stretch in your back until it almost makes contact with your chest.

Hold this position for a count, then return slowly back to the starting position.

Repeat for as many reps and sets as desired and switch with the opposite arms.

Deadlift

Start off standing in front of a barbell with your feet shoulder-width apart.

Grab the barbell with a shoulder width grip, overhand. Keep your head up and your back straight. Do not round your back.

Pick up the barbell while keeping your arms extended straight down and keeping the barbell close to your legs as if you were dragging it up your legs. Do not round your back.

Stand up straight with the barbell in your hands, and refrain from moving your arms.

Bend back down at the knees with barbell and place on the floor.

Deadlift with Dumbbells

Start off standing in front of a pair of dumbbells with your feet shoulder-width apart.

Grab the dumbbells with a shoulder width grip, overhand. Keep your head up and your back straight. Do not round your back.

Pick up the dumbbells while keeping your arms extended straight down and keeping the dumbbells close to your legs as if you were dragging it up your legs.

Stand up straight with the dumbbells in your hands, and refrain from moving your arms.

Bend back down at the knees with dumbbells and place on the floor.

Band Row

Start by wrapping up a band around a pole or door handle and grab the band handle with both hands in an overhand grip.

Keep your knees slightly bent and back straight, pull the handle in towards your midsection, keeping your elbows at your sides, squeeze with your back and hold for a count.

Return back to the starting position.

Legs

Barbell Squat

With the weighted barbell resting in a power rack or on a set of squat stands step under the bar.

Position your body so that the barbell is touching your upper back or traps, keeping your chest up, head facing forward and your feet shoulder width apart.

Grab the bar, palms facing to the front.

Step back once or far enough so that you clear the rack, but not too far.

Keeping your body as upright as possible and looking forward squat all the way down until your legs are just to parallel. Keep your weight even on both legs.

Hold for a count then drive your weight up as you return back to the starting position.

Note:

Do not let your knees go passed your toes or cave in when you squat down. Have someone looking to make sure or squat in front of a mirror.

Dumbbell Squat

Start off standing in front of a pair of dumbbells with your feet shoulder-width apart.

Grab the dumbbells with a overhand grip so that the dumbbells are at your sides.

Keeping your body as upright as possible and looking forward squat all the way down until your legs are just to parallel. Keep your weight even on both legs.

Hold for 1 count then drive your weight up as you return back to the starting position.

Note:

Do not let your knees go passed your toes or cave in when you squat down. Have someone looking to make sure or squat in front of a mirror.

Band Leg Extensions

Secure one end of the band underneath a chair or bench and secure the other band on one ankle.

Extend your leg straight by straighten your knee,

Return to starting position.

Repeat this sequence on the other leg.

Machine Leg Extensions

Sit in the seat after you adjust it to your body type.

Position both ankles under the pads.

Select the proper weight.

Extend your legs straight with the dumbbell by straighten your knee,

Return to starting position.

Legs: Hamstrings and Buttocks

Bridges

Lie on your back with your knees bent and feet placed flat on the floor.

Place your hands out to your sides and lift your hips up until your thighs and trunk form a straight line.

Slowly return to the starting position.

These are just a small sample of exercises that you can easily perform to start or resume your training program. The important thing is to choose a few exercises for each body part. Also, it is very important to perform all movements correctly with the proper form before adding weight.

For example, if you perform the bench press do so with little to no weight on the bar until you learn the proper way to perform the movement. If you need more instruction on how to perform an exercise there are excellent resources on the internet that you can look at.

Cooldown

After your training session it is important you let your slowly ramp down from your workout. A five to ten-minute cool down will allow your blood flow and heart rate return to their normal levels. A cool down can consist of light aerobic activity such as jogging, stretching, or just walking is sufficient.

CHAPTER 6

Gym Membership vs Home Gym

n the last section we talked about some of the equipment you can use to train with. Also, we discussed and what exercises you can use to start your training program in order to look great and get stronger. Now you need somewhere to perform those exercises. Next, we're going to discuss the pros and cons of a gym membership verses training at home.

Gym

Basically, you could get stronger anywhere by using your bodyweight or whatever you can find as a means of resistance.

However, to progressively build and challenge your muscles you'll need more resistance and equipment options than what may available. You can solve this by becoming a member of a gym or fitness center.

Now when I say gym, this means a facility that has adequate space, equipment, and flooring that requires some sort of payment to use the facility. This could include a commercially operated gym, a community center, the Y, a corporate wellness center or anything similar.

Finding a good gym to meet your goals can be a challenge. However, when you do find one it will be a great asset. There are advantages and disadvantages to working out in a gym:

Disadvantages

Access to equipment.

You wouldn't be the only person in the gym. You'd have to share equipment and sometimes wait, taking up your allotted training time.

Gyms can be intimidating.

If you're a beginner a gym with lots of equipment can be overwhelming.

If you're a beginner a gym with lots of people can be overwhelming.

If you're a woman you may have to deal with guys staring at you.

Money factor.

Depending on the facility you may have to pay for services you will not use such as a pool, hot tub, or daycare.

Advantages

Meet new people.

> You can meet people with similar fitness goals and fitness levels.

More equipment.

> Most gyms have plenty of equipment, more so than a typical home gym setup.

> You have many options of equipment to train on barbells, machines, etc.

> You wouldn't get bored performing the same workouts or movements.

Change of scenery.

> Sometimes it's nice to get out of the house and train somewhere else.

More Room.

> Training in a spacious venue like a gym can provide more options for training.

Home Gym

A home gym is self-explanatory. This means you train at your place of residence with whatever equipment you can obtain. Also, this option not only includes your dwelling but the park, a friend's home, or even a playground.

Advantages

Freedom to train when you want.

You can choose when and how long to train with no time restrictions.

Better concentration.

You can concentrate on your workout with little no people interfering with your training.

Equipment.

You choose what equipment is important to you for your needs.

No fees.

A monthly or yearly fee can be expensive and eat in to your budget.

Disadvantages

Obtaining equipment is costly.

Assembling a wish list or all the equipment you need can be expensive.

Limited equipment.

> Space in your home is limited, so you can only have so much equipment to train with.

Potential distractions.

Many things could interfere with training, dog, visitors, children etc.

As you can see training to strengthen your body is not difficult. It just takes planning and effort. It doesn't matter if you're a member of a full-service fitness center or you're doing bodyweight squats or push-ups in the park, you have the tools and information to transform your body.

CHAPTER 7

Training Journal

When someone embarks on a long journey, they capture the moments they experience as memories to look back on. These days travelers usually take photos or capture moments by video. In the days before electronics a traveler would record their voyage in a book or journal which would later remind them of important aspects of the trip such as events that happened, their experiences, what went wrong and the things that went well.

As you start your journey for a stronger, healthier body, it is imperative that you keep a journal. This will enable you record important aspects of your fitness journey.

Recording important training information such as the weight you used, the number of sets and repetitions you completed, and the exercises and movements you performed will come into play when you want to advance your program or track your progress. Keeping a journal will help you make adjustments to your program if you are not seeing the results you should.

However, a lot of people do not keep training journals. They don't see the value behind it. They leave it up to their memory which can falter. The last thing you want to do is try to remember how many reps you did after an exhausting set of squats.

Or after a 45-minute workout trying to remember the sets and reps of the exercise you completed. What will happen is that you'll keeping doing the same workout over and over again and wonder why you're not making any progress.

What type of journal or log should you use?

You can use anything from an elaborate hardbound journal to a spiral notebook. The important thing is that you record your training. You can use a computer, a spreadsheet, your cell phone or whatever. The important thing is that you record your training. There are even websites where you can create an account and record your workouts using a wearable fitness tracker. Some trackers are smart enough to detect your motion and count repetitions for certain movement patterns.

Things you should record in your journal

Below is a list of common items to record in your journal. However, you can record just about anything you what if you feel it's important to you and has value when you review it later.

Strength training:

Goals

Sets

Repetitions

Weight used

Day

Time

Location

Equipment

Training cycle

Shoes you wore

Clothes you wore

Training partner

Rest time

Environment

How you felt

What you ate before and after

Training program

Aches and pains

For other activities such as running, swimming, yoga etc.:

Distance

Pace

Terrain

Drills

Laps

Location

Rest days

Events

Stretching

Body weight

Heart rate

Progression

State of mind

Travel

CHAPTER 8

Recovery, Overtraining, and Muscle Soreness

Strength training involves putting forth maximum effort in order to receive the results you want. You must be committed to consistency and doing the little things daily. However too much of a good thing can backfire and cause more harm than good.

Strength training presents stresses to the body and its various systems. Strength training done without proper planning can lead to your body exceeding its rate of adapting to the stress placed upon it. This can lead to excessive training including overreaching and overtraining.

Excessive training.

Excessive training refers to training where the number of exercises, sets, or reps are increased without proper progression. Also, excessive training refers to the intensity of training that is increased too rapidly and without proper planning for its increase. When you're in this state, you experience no additional improvement in conditioning or performance. This can lead to a chronic state of fatigue.

 If you are training too often, for example daily, your muscles become chronically depleted of their energy reserves and the body undergoes inflammation in response to this training[44].

The stress of excessive training can exceed the body's ability to recover and adapt, which results in more catabolism (breakdown) than anabolism (build up).

Because each person is different, people will experience varied levels of fatigue during repeated days and weeks of training, so not all situations can be classified as excessive training[44].

Overreaching

Overreaching happens when the physical and mental stress training results in a decrease in a person's ability to exercise and perform over a short time period. This is when you're not feeling up to exercising and feel kind of drained[45].

Recovering from this state may take several days to several weeks. This condition is often mistakenly referred to as overtraining[44,45].

Overtraining

Overtraining is related to overreaching however it is not the same. Overtraining occurs when the physical and mental stress of training results in a decrease in a person's ability to exercise and perform over a long time period. This is more than feeling kind of tired. This is chronic fatigue or nagging injuries that stops you from training and exercise. Recovering from this state may take several weeks to several months[44,45].

Several mental and physical events can contribute to overreaching such as:

Not taking enough rest days between training.

Not eating enough nutrients.

Doing too many exercises in one workout.

Too much training frequency

Too much training intensity

Too much training volume

Aging

Poorly designed equipment

Family problems

Excessive heat or cold

Schedule conflicts

Anger

Financial status

Personality conflicts

Fatigue that often follows one or more exhaustive training sessions is usually corrected by a few days of rest coupled with a carbohydrate rich diet. Overtraining, on the other hand, is characterized by a sudden decline in performance that cannot be remedied by a few days of rest and dietary manipulation.

Muscle soreness

As you train your body will undergo the processes of inflammation, repair, and remodeling in response to the training stress.

This will lead to a certain degree of muscle soreness or   pain which you may be experienced after a workout.

The muscle soreness that you experience directly after a workout is known as acute muscle soreness. The muscle soreness that your body experiences after 12 to 48 hours after strenuous exercise is known as delayed onset muscle soreness (DOMS)[46].

There are several theories on the cause muscle soreness and inflammation. One theory asserts that it may be due to a reduction in blood flow to the muscle and an accumulation of metabolic byproducts like hydrogen ions or lactic acid[46].

Avoiding Excessive Training, Overreaching, and Overtraining.

Can you avoid excessive training, overreaching, and overtraining? Yes, however not by not training, but by managing your training and managing the repeated stress over time you put your muscles, bones, tendons, and nerves through during training which is part of your physical and physiological well-being. You can avoid these conditions in several ways:

Using proper lifting form and techniques when training.

Managing your training methods such as sets and reps.

Using recovery techniques such as meditation, visualization, foam rolling, and massage techniques[47].

Managing all other stressors in your life that can interfere with your training such as environmental, psychological, sociological, biochemical, physiological.

Getting proper sleep and rest.

However, one of the best ways to minimize the risk of overtraining is to follow cyclic training procedures and alternating easy, moderate and hard periods of training, also known as periodization.

Periodization

Periodization is a way to plan and schedule your training, usually over the long term. It involves dividing your training into segments or cycles, balancing periods of low intensity with high intensity with the goal of improving your strength fitness level

Your periodization plan is the breakdown of your training plan and goals which can be divided into the following three training phases or cycles:

Overall Training Cycle

This is the period from when you decide to train for a goal until the deadline of that goal. Basically, you are preparing your body for some type of an event. This training period is usually a considerable amount of time, months, sometimes even a year or more. For some athletes it is not uncommon to have cycles consisting of multiple years.

During this cycle you will complete multiple types of training protocols to prepare your body for your goal. Training protocols such as strength, speed, sports skills, mobility etc.

For example, if you're preparing for a running event such as a 10K or marathon or you're training for a strength event such as weightlifting you'll spend several weeks or months on these training protocols. It all depends on your training goals, your level or fitness, and your deadline date. This cycle is sometimes referred to as a macrocycle.

Medium Training Cycle

A medium training cycle is multiple divisions of an overall training cycle. This is where you'll work or train on a particular area of fitness or sport such as general fitness, strength, or mobility. This cycle is sometimes referred to as a mesocycle.

Small Training Cycle

A small training cycle is described as one time period of intensity. Periods of high intensity must be followed by periods of low intensity or rest before another period of high intensity can occur. For certain muscles or muscle groups, this could take as little as few days and as much as several weeks. This cycle is sometimes referred to as a microcycle.

For example, let's say you're preparing for an event scheduled for September and your overall cycle is one year. You can divide that in four time periods consisting of three months which would be your medium training cycle and divide that into multiple training periods which is your small training cycle.

Overall Cycle: One Year			
Medium Cycle	Medium Cycle	Medium Cycle	Medium Cycle
Small Cycles	Small Cycles	Small Cycles	Small Cycles

Your small training cycle then could consist of each month in the medium cycle. Then you can break the small cycle down further into weeks or days.

Think of your periodization schedule like stairs in a tall building. Think of the entire building, from the first floor to the roof, as an overall training cycle or macrocycle. Each flight of stairs to each floor is the medium training cycle or mesocycle. And each step is a small training cycle or microcycle. You need to take each step to get to your goal at the top. Trying to jump steps will more than likely result in injury. It's a long process that takes patience and effort but it will pay off when you reach the top.

During a training cycle there will be times when the amount of weight you lift during a workout is decreased. This is usually referred to as a deload training session and involves a scaled down training session or sometimes complete and total rest.

There is a reason why sports and athletes at every level incorporate a periodization cycle and have an off season. It's to let the body recovery from the previous season and get ready for the upcoming season. Periodization helps, not prevents, but helps prevent injuries.

Recovery

When you were younger you recovered quickly from training, even intense training. However, as you age recovery becomes more important to your, fitness, strength, overall health goals.

You can't train 365 days and expect to stay healthy and functional. Your body needs time away from the stress of training and it needs methods to heal it. Left to its own devices your body will do that by itself, however it will take a very long time, longer than you want. This means that as the level and difficulty of your training increases, you must pay even more attention to rest and recovery.

In addition to sleep and nutrition there are many forms of recovery, including various types of bodywork that are available:

Chiropractic adjustments

Massage

Whirlpool

Sauna

Acupressure

Acupuncture

Self-massage using a foam roller, tennis ball, or a product called a Thera Cane

Ice, applied to muscles and joints

Heat, applied to muscles

Anti-inflammatories

Leg elevation

Compression devices

Contrast Showers. This consist of alternating between hot and cold burst of water for 1-2 minutes increments 4-6 times following a workout.

If you don't incorporate recovery into your training you won't be able to overload the body enough to cause growth and progress. Over a lifetime of training your body will decrease in its recovery ability, however during that lifetime it will also undergo certain training effects that will allow for harder and more frequent training.

Phillip J Germany II

102

CHAPTER 9

Nutrition

Nutrition is not complicated. If you want to have energy, decrease body fat, look great, and feel your best then you have a pretty good idea of what to eat and what not to eat.

It recommended that you stay away from the following:

Foods that contain artificial colors, sulfates, nitrates, and preservatives.

High Fructose Corn Syrup.

Processed meats with preservatives and nitrates.

Trans Fats. Foods with shortenings, hydrogenated oils like margarine.

Unhealthy fats that are processed and cause inflammation such as products labeled vegetable oil such as palm, cottonseed, corn, or soy oil.

Stressing over the foods you eat, how you train, how to lose weight will not help you. All of the confusion and frustration that involves what to eat no longer needs to be a part of your life.

More importantly, getting rid of this stress can actually improve your weight loss and overall health. Worrying over what you eat can actually cause excessive psychological stress making gaining strength more difficult.

Below we're going to focus on macronutrients carbohydrates, proteins, and fats. Water, by some, is considered a fourth macronutrient. It provides no energy to the body however it is very essential.

Carbohydrates

Carbohydrates are used by your body as fuel for several functions including your brain and muscle protein synthesis which is needed for your muscles to grow. Carbohydrates are also used to fuel your training. When you eat carbohydrates, they enter the body and turns into glucose which circulates in the blood stream. When carbohydrates are stored in the body they are referred to as glycogen.

Glycogen is stored in three places, your liver, fat cells, and muscles. Any excess carbohydrates that can't be stored in the liver or muscles are stored in fat cells, which you don't want and is counterproductive to your strength training and health.

When you are training hard, the glycogen in your muscles are called upon to give you the fuel needed to train. So, carbohydrates are important to becoming strong. To minimize body fat accumulation, you should eat your carbs in the form of vegetables, fruits, and certain grains.

Protein

If you want to build strength, muscle, and look and feel great protein is a must. Protein is not stored in the body however like carbs and fat. However, if you eat excess protein, more than your body needs at one time, it will be converted into fat.

According to some research older active adults need more protein to overcome muscle loss to Sarcopenia[48]. Red meat, poultry, seafood, and eggs are all good sources. Plant sources such as beans, unprocessed soy, nuts, seeds, and vegetables are excellent also.

Fat

Contrary to what you've heard or read in the past fat is not bad and will not increase your body fat. It's the excess of calories over and above what your body burns and uses for energy that will make you fat. So, your body needs fat for many functions and processes including fuel.

Fat, sometimes referred to as lipids, provides energy for your body at rest and during exercise. However, during intense strength training fat is not as efficient. Needless to say, fat should not be avoided under any circumstances. Its rich in vitamins and minerals that support a healthy body and an active lifestyle. Healthy sources of fat include olive, coconut, and avocado oil, nuts, nut oils, and omega-3 oils.

Water

Water is needed for life. As mentioned, water is considered by some as a macronutrient. It's essential for optimum health in addition to muscle protein synthesis. There are guidelines but the amount of water you need depends on your activity level, body size, and climate. So, if you're running, working construction, or working in a steel plant in July, you'll need more water than if you're working in an office in April or sitting at home in January.

However, you should not wait until you're thirsty to hydrate. Hydrating means drinking water or getting water from foods or even tea. Soda, diet soda, and other sugary drinks are counterproductive and should not count in your water budget.

Bottomline

If you eat less calories than you burn and eat nutrient dense foods you can still eat the foods you enjoy and preserve your strength and lean body mass while you lose body fat. You'll be better off in the long run and you will greatly increase your chances of keeping the fat off. By being flexible about eating and not overly restrictive it allows you to enact a great deal of dietary restraint without feeling deprived or bored of your food choices.

CHAPTER 10

Sleep

Sleep is not only an integral part of life but also an integral part of the recovery process from training. All of the training, workouts, and exercises you do are futile if you don't get the proper sleep.

The anabolic processes which occur during sleep benefits not only your normal body maintenance but also your strength building. Your anabolic hormones such Testosterone and Human Growth Hormone (HGH) are secreted during sleep. So, in order to optimize and balance your hormones a good night's sleep is a must. At least seven hours is the target for sleep[49,50].

As people age, they tend to have trouble getting to or stay sleep. This constant interruption hampers your REM (Rapid Eye Movement) sleep cycles. REM sleep occurs at intervals during the night and is characterized by rapid eye movements, more dreaming, body movement, faster pulse, and faster breathing. You need deep REM sleep in order for our anabolic hormones to stay elevated longer.

However, many things can rob you of a full night's sleep. Things such as anxiety, stress, medications, muscle and joint pain, alcohol or caffeine, and for men excessive urination due to prostate problems.

Some of these issues can be handle by lifestyle modification, holistic methods, or medical treatment[50].

Eating a big meal too close to bed time can interrupt your sleep also. When digestion takes place your body temperature increases thus causing a delay or stifling the body's production of HGH[51].

Also, the types of foods you eat near bedtime can have an effect. Foods containing chocolate, high fats, and spicy foods can interrupt your sleep[51].

If you have trouble sleeping a sleep study can revel conditions such as sleep apnea. Sleep apnea is a common disorder in which you have one or more pauses in breathing or shallow breaths while you sleep.

Many large, muscular men have sleep apnea that can easily be treated with a CPAP device that not only will improve sleep quality and performance, but can lower blood pressure and greatly improve overall health[50].

Why We Need Sleep
We need sleep for obvious reasons such as resting our bodies and allowing our biological processes to take place during the night. However, there are more reasons why living beings sleep. Here are four theories[51,52].

1) The Adaptive Theory

This theory says that sleep improves the likelihood of survival. Those with sleeping habits appropriate to their environment are most likely to survive. Nocturnal species have very different sleep habits than diurnal hunters, for example, making them more likely to flourish. So, this is why your cat is up all night, and you are awake all day. It's about survival[52].

2) The Information Consolidation Theory

The information consolidation theory of sleep is based on cognitive research and suggests that people sleep in order to process information that has been acquired during the day. In addition to processing information from the day prior, this theory also argues that sleep allows the brain to prepare for the day to come[51].

3) The Restorative Theory

According to this theory, the body restores itself during sleep. Researchers know that neurotoxins are neutralized during sleep and have reported that cells divide, tissue synthesizes, and growth hormones are released during slow-wave sleep. Athletes, for example, spend more time in slow-wave sleep than others, and children and young people spend a larger portion of their sleep in slow-wave sleep than older people[51,52].

4) The Programming-Reprogramming or Brain Theory

This theory states that unimportant information is erased from memory and important information is locked into more permanent memory. Infants, who are acquiring information at a rate faster than at any other point during life, sleep most. Also, neural reorganization and growth of the brain's structure and function occurs. Brain cells produce waste products which needs disposal and happens during sleep[53].

Getting Better Sleep

In order to get optimal sleep, examine your sleeping environment and pay attention to the following:

Room Temperature

Be sure that the room you sleep in is on the cool side.

Bedding

Make sure your bedding isn't causing you harm such as allergenic materials. Make sure you get it as comfortable as you can make it.

Quiet

Make sure it's quiet. Traffic noise, barking dogs, and loud neighbors will make sleep impossible. Use ear muffs or ear plugs if you can't get rid of the noise.

White Noise

Some people find that white noise such as a constant drone helps. You can use a soft sound device or app that makes noise such as a flowing stream, wind, or rain.

Rise Time

Get up at the same time every morning, even after a bad night's sleep. The next night, you'll be sleepy at bedtime.

Stay Up

If you wake up in the middle of the night and can't fall back to sleep, get out of bed and return only when you are sleepy.

Sleep When Sleepy

Don't go to bed until you're sleepy. If you have trouble sleeping, try going to bed later or getting up earlier.

Miscellaneous

Avoid worrying, watching TV, reading scary books, and doing other things in bed besides sleeping, and sex.

Darkness

You might think your room is dark enough for sleep but it may not be. Lights from your electronic devices, neighbor, or even moon light can become a nuisance. Your room should be dark enough so you can't see anything. Use blackout shades, towels, cardboard, blankets, anything that will make your room dark.

Create a Bedtime Ritual

You can actually train yourself to get sleepy at the same time every night by creating some sleep associations. Changing into pajamas, reading a book, listening to relaxing music, are things that tell your body its bedtime.

Meditation or Visualization

To release the stress of your day. Once you are in bed and the lights are out, you can imagine leaving all of your worries and concerns.

Sleep Aids

There are sleep aids such as medication or supplements that can help you fall asleep and stay asleep. Constant use of these aids can be problematic and may do more harm than good if not used judiciously or monitored by a doctor. However, sleep aids should be used in extreme cases and only temporarily. Over-the-counter agents such as Melatonin and Valerian and prescription sleep aids can also help. However, be advised, any type of pharmacologic sleep aid over-the-counter or prescription should be under a doctor's supervision.

Conclusion

This book is a starting point on your journey to a strong healthy body that will stand up to the unforgiving process of aging. When I wrote this book, I wanted it to be a helpful source for beginners to start their journey to strength training. I'm confident this book will help you break through the confusion of starting a path to a stronger body. You only get one body.

Sarcopenia is serious. It can lead to a frail and sick body and it can slowly appear over time if it's not addressed. You will never solve a problem if you only address the symptoms. You must address the causes as well. Healthy aging and staving off sarcopenia involve building muscle and growing stronger, and the best way to accomplish this is strength training. Instead of withering away in your advanced years you can build muscle, making you bold and strong, giving you the freedom to feel and look the way you want. Good luck!

Phillip J Germany II

114

Appendix

7-Day Food Log

7-Day Training Journal

Phillip J Germany II

7-Day Food Log and Training Log

The purpose this log is to quantify your food normal intake. So do not alter your eating habits in any way. It is important that this record be both accurate and representative of your normal dietary intake.

You don't have to be neurotic about it but it's important that you record every single item that you consume (this includes fluids, condiments, etc.)

The log is designed for 4 meals a day. This includes snacks. So, for example if you eat cheese and crackers 2 hours before your dinner that's considered a meal.

In the quantity column record the amount you ate. For example, 6 crackers and 2 slices of cheese. If you want to use a food scale or measuring cups to obtain a precision amount of your food that's up to you. For this purpose, it's not required. If you need extra space just use the notes section.

The bottom line is just write down the foods things you eat.

For the training log write down the time, date, type of workout, and the things you did during your workout.

And when you want to continue to record your training pick up a copy of *Too Strong to Grow Old 90-Day Training Journal* and use it as a companion to this book.

FOOD	QUANTITY
MEAL 1	
MEAL 2	
MEAL 3	
MEAL 4	

FOOD	QUANTITY
MEAL 1	
MEAL 2	
MEAL 3	
MEAL 4	

FOOD	QUANTITY
MEAL 1	
MEAL 2	
MEAL 3	
MEAL 4	

FOOD	QUANTITY
MEAL 1	
MEAL 2	
MEAL 3	
MEAL 4	

FOOD	QUANTITY
MEAL 1	
MEAL 2	
MEAL 3	
MEAL 4	

FOOD	QUANTITY
MEAL 1	
MEAL 2	
MEAL 3	
MEAL 4	

FOOD	QUANTITY
MEAL 1	
MEAL 2	
MEAL 3	
MEAL 4	

7-Day Training Log

DATE: / /   **M   T   W   TH   F   S   SU**

TIME: **START:**   **END:**

TYPE OF WORKOUT:

Strength Training

Cardio

Yoga

Other:

WORKOUT DETAILS:

NOTES:

DATE: / /   M   T   W   TH   F   S   SU

TIME: **START:**   **END:**

TYPE OF WORKOUT:

Strength Training

Cardio

Yoga

Other:

WORKOUT DETAILS:

NOTES:

DATE: / /   **M**   **T**   **W**   **TH**   **F**   **S**   **SU**

TIME: **START:**   **END:**

TYPE OF WORKOUT:

Strength Training

Cardio

Yoga

Other:

WORKOUT DETAILS:

NOTES:

DATE: / /   M   T   W   TH   F   S   SU

TIME: **START:**   **END:**

TYPE OF WORKOUT:

Strength Training

Cardio

Yoga

Other:

WORKOUT DETAILS:

NOTES:

DATE: / /   M   T   W   TH   F   S   SU

TIME: START: END:

TYPE OF WORKOUT:

Strength Training

Cardio

Yoga

Other:

WORKOUT DETAILS:

NOTES:

DATE: / /   M   T   W   TH   F   S   SU

TIME: START: END:

TYPE OF WORKOUT:

Strength Training

Cardio

Yoga

Other:

WORKOUT DETAILS:

NOTES:

DATE: / /   **M**   **T**   **W**   **TH**   **F**   **S**   **SU**

TIME: **START:**   **END:**

TYPE OF WORKOUT:

Strength Training

Cardio

Yoga

Other:

WORKOUT DETAILS:

NOTES:

Phillip J Germany II

REFERENCES

1. Chishti, Hakim, *The Traditional Healer's Handbook. Vermont: Healing Arts Press. 1988 p. 11.*

2. Mason, Caitlin et al. "Influence of diet, exercise, and serum vitamin d on sarcopenia in postmenopausal women." *Medicine and science in sports and exercise* vol. 45,4 (2013): 607-14. doi:10.1249/MSS.0b013e31827aa3fa

3. Akın, S., Mucuk, S., Öztürk, A. *et al.* Muscle function-dependent sarcopenia and cut-off values of possible predictors in community-dwelling Turkish elderly: calf circumference, midarm muscle circumference and walking speed. *Eur J Clin Nutr* **69,** 1087–1090 (2015). https://doi.org/10.1038/ejcn.2015.42

4. Schoenfeld, Brad J, Journal of Strength and Conditioning Research: October 2010 - Volume 24 - Issue 10 - p 2857-2872 doi: 10.1519/JSC.0b013e3181e840f3

5. Karsten Keller, Martin Engelhardt, Strength and muscle mass loss with aging process. Age and strength loss, Muscles, Ligaments and Tendons Journal 2013; 346 3 (4): 346-350.

6. Melov S., Tarnopolsky M.A., Beckman K., Felkey K., and Hubbard A. (2007) Resistance Exercise Reverses Aging in Human Skeletal Muscle. PLoS ONE 2(5): e465.

7. Lin, Tzu-Wei, and Yu-Min Kuo. "Exercise benefits brain function: the monoamine connection." *Brain sciences* vol. 3,1 39-53. 11 Jan. 2013, doi:10.3390/brainsci3010039

8. *The Journals of Gerontology: Series A*, Volume 50A, Issue Special Issue, November 1995, Pages 147–150.

9. LEMMER, JEFFREY T.; IVEY, FREDERICK M.; RYAN, ALICE S.; MARTEL, GREG F.; HURLBUT, DIANE E.; METTER, JEFFREY E.; FOZARD, JAMES L.; FLEG, JEROME L.; HURLEY, BEN F. Effect of strength training on resting metabolic rate and physical activity: age and gender comparisons, Medicine and Science in Sports and Exercise: April 2001 - Volume 33 - Issue 4 - p 532-541

10. FEIGENBAUM, MATTHEW S.; POLLOCK, MICHAEL L. Prescription of resistance training for health and disease, Medicine & Science in Sports & Exercise: January 1999 - Volume 31 - Issue 1 - p 38-45.

11. Stanton AM, Handy AB, Meston CM. The Effects of Exercise on Sexual Function in Women. Sex Med Rev 2018; 6:548–557.

12. Stanghelle B[1], Bentzen H[2], Giangregorio L[3], Pripp AH[4], Skelton D[5], Bergland A[6].
Effects of a resistance and balance exercise program on physical fitness, health-related quality of life and fear of falling in older women with osteoporosis and vertebral fracture: a randomized controlled trial. Osteoporosis Int. 2020 Jan 10. doi: 10.1007/s00198-019-05256-4.

13. Lee, In-Hee, and Sang-Young Park. "Balance improvement by strength training for the elderly." *Journal of physical therapy science* vol. 25,12 (2013): 1591-3. doi:10.1589/jpts.25.1591

14.O'Connor, P.J., Herring, M.P. and Carvalho, A. (2010). Mental health benefits of strength training in adults. American Journal of Lifestyle Medicine, 4(5), 377-396.

15. Sun, Fei et al. "Physical activity in older people: a systematic review." *BMC public health* vol. 13 449. 6 May. 2013, doi:10.1186/1471-2458-13-449.

16. Anton, Stephen D et al. "Successful aging: Advancing the science of physical independence in older adults." *Ageing research reviews* vol. 24,Pt B (2015): 304-27. doi:10.1016/j.arr.2015.09.005.

17. Tavoian, Dallin et al. "A Randomized Clinical Trial Comparing Three Different Exercise Strategies for Optimizing Aerobic Capacity and Skeletal Muscle Performance in Older Adults: Protocol for the DART Study." *Frontiers in medicine* vol. 6 236. 22 Oct. 2019, doi:10.3389/fmed.2019.00236.

18. Shaw, B S, and I Shaw. "Compatibility of concurrent aerobic and resistance training on maximal aerobic capacity in sedentary males." *Cardiovascular journal of Africa* vol. 20,2 (2009): 104-6.

19. Sukwon Kim, Thurmon Lockhart, Karen Roberto, The effects of 8-week balance training or weight training: For the elderly on fear of falling measures and social activity levels., Qual Ageing. 2009 November 20; 10(4): 37–48.

20. Gómez-Cabello A , Ara I, González-Agüero A, Casajús JA, Vicente-Rodríguez G. Effects of training on bone mass in older

adults: a systematic review. Sports Med. 2012 Apr 1;42(4):301-25. doi: 10.2165/11597670-000000000-00000.

21. A Ram Hong, Sang Wan Kim, Effects of Resistance Exercise on Bone Health, Endocrinol Metabolism 2018;33:435-444.

22. Liu Y, Lee DC, Zhu Y, et al. Associations of resistance exercise with cardiovascular disease, morbidity, and mortality [pubished online October 29, 2018]. *Med Sci Sports Exerc.* 2018; doi: 10.1249/MSS.0000000000001822.

23. https://www.ajmc.com/newsroom/a-little-weight-training-can-do-a-lot-to-cut-cardiovascular-risk-study-finds.

24. Hunter, G.R., McCarthy, J.P. & Bamman, M.M. Effects of Resistance Training on Older Adults. *Sports Med* **34,** 329–348 (2004).

25. www.cdc.gov/chronicdisease/resources/publications/ factsheets/arthritis.

26. Liu-Ambrose, T.Y.L., Khan, K.M., Eng, J.J. *et al.* Both resistance and agility training reduce back pain and improve health-related quality of life in older women with low bone mass. *Osteoporosis Int* **16,** 1321–1329 (2005)

27. Danneels LA, Vanderstraeten GG, Cambier DC, *et al* Effects of three different training modalities on the cross-sectional area of the lumbar multifidus muscle in patients with chronic low back pain

British Journal of Sports Medicine 2001; **35:186**-191.

28. Fleck, S.J., Falkel, J.E. Value of Resistance Training for the Reduction of Sports Injuries. *Sports Medicine* 3, 61–68 (1986).

29. Mei-Hwa Jan, Jiu-Jeng Lin, Jiann-Jong Liau, Yeong-Fwu Lin, Da-Hon Lin,_Investigation of Clinical Effects of High- and Low-Resistance Training for Patients With Knee Osteoarthritis: A Randomized Controlled Trial, *Physical Therapy*, Volume 88, Issue 4, 1 April 2008, Pages 427–436.

30.https://orthoinfo.aaos.org/en/recovery/knee-conditioning-program

31. Baechle, T.R. and R.W. Earle. *Essentials of Strength Training and Conditioning*, 3rd ed. Champaign, IL: Human Kinetics. 2008.

32. Schoenfeld, Brad. *The Science and Development of Muscle Hypertrophy,* 1st ed. Champaign, IL: Human Kinetics. 2016.

33. Keller, Karsten and Engelhardt, Martin. *Strength and muscle mass loss with aging process, age and strength loss,* Muscles, Ligaments and Tendons Journal 2013; (4): 346-350.

34. Kumar, V, Selby, A, Rankin, D, Patel, R, Atherton, P. Age related differences in the dose response relationship of muscle protein synthesis to resistance exercise in young and old men. *J Physiol.* 587: 211-217, 2009.

35. MICHAEL H. THOMAS, STEVE P. BURNS, Increasing Lean Mass and Strength: A Comparison of High Frequency Strength Training to Lower Frequency Strength Training, International Journal of Exercise Science 9(2): 159-167, 2016.

36. Easthope, C.S., Hausswirth, C., Louis, J. *et al.* Effects of a trail running competition on muscular performance and efficiency in well-trained young and master athletes. *Eur J Appl Physiol* **110,** 1107–1116 (2010). https://doi.org/10.1007/s00421-010-1597-1

37. Sultana, F., Abbiss, C.R., Louis, J. *et al.* Age-related changes in cardio-respiratory responses and muscular performance following an Olympic triathlon in well-trained triathletes. *Eur J Appl Physiol* 112, 1549–1556 (2012).

38. https://www.medicalnewstoday.com/articles/145855#management

39. Rob D Herbert, Michael Gabriel, Effects of stretching before and after exercising on muscle soreness and risk of injury: systematic review; BMJ VOLUME 325 31 AUGUST 2002

40. Mayer F, Scharhag-Rosenberger F, Carlsohn A, et al.: The intensity and effects of strength training in the elderly. Dtsch Arztebl Int 2011; 108(21): 359–64.

41. Rubini, E.C., Costa, A.L.L. & Gomes, P.S.C. The Effects of Stretching on Strength Performance. *Sports Med* **37,** 213–224 (2007).

42. Walsh, Greg, Effect of static and dynamic muscle stretching as part of warm up procedures on knee joint proprioception and strength, <u>Human Movement Science</u> <u>Volume 55</u>, October 2017, Pages 189-195.

43. Paoli A, Gentil P, Moro T, Marcolin G and Bianco A (2017) Resistance Training with Single vs. Multi-joint Exercises at Equal Total Load Volume: Effects on Body Composition, Cardiorespiratory Fitness, and Muscle Strength. *Front. Physiol.* 8:1105. doi: 10.3389/fphys.2017.01105

44. Kreher, Jeffrey B, and Jennifer B Schwartz. "Overtraining syndrome: a practical guide." *Sports health* vol. 4,2 (2012): 128-38. doi:10.1177/1941738111434406.

45. Halson, S.L., Jeukendrup, A.E. Does Overtraining Exist? *Sports Med* **34,** 967–981 (2004).

46. Dupuy, Olivier et al. "An Evidence-Based Approach for Choosing Post-exercise Recovery Techniques to Reduce Markers of Muscle Damage, Soreness, Fatigue, and Inflammation: A Systematic Review With Meta-Analysis." *Frontiers in physiology* vol. 9 403. 26 Apr. 2018, doi:10.3389/fphys.2018.00403

47. Pearcey, Gregory E P et al. "Foam rolling for delayed-onset muscle soreness and recovery of dynamic performance

measures." *Journal of athletic training* vol. 50,1 (2015): 5-13. doi:10.4085/1062-6050-50.1.01

48. Wayne W. Campbell, Todd A. Trappe, Robert R. Wolfe, William J. Evans, The Recommended Dietary Allowance for Protein May Not Be Adequate for Older People to Maintain Skeletal Muscle, *The Journals of Gerontology: Series A*, Volume 56, Issue 6, 1 June 2001, Pages M373–M380,

49. https://www.cdc.gov/media/releases/2016/p0215-enough-sleep.html

50. Brinkman JE, Sharma S. Physiology, Sleep. [Updated 2019 Mar 16]. In: StatPearls [Internet]. Treasure Island (FL): StatPearls Publishing; 2020 Jan

51. Kinsey, Amber W, and Michael J Ormsbee. "The health impact of nighttime eating: old and new perspectives." *Nutrients* vol. 7,4 2648-62. 9 Apr. 2015, doi:10.3390/nu7042648.

52. Ezenwanne E. Current concepts in the neurophysiologic basis of sleep; a review. *Ann Med Health Sci Res*. 2011;1(2):173–179.

53. Xie L, Kang H, Xu Q, et al. Sleep drives metabolite clearance from the adult brain. *Science*. 2013;342(6156):373–377.
54. Verkhoshansky, Y. and M. Siff. Supertraining, 6th Edition: Expanded Version. SSTM. 2009.

55. McGinnis, P. *Biomechanics of Sport and Exercise*. 3rd ed. Champaign, IL: Human Kinetics. 2013.

56. Schoenfeld, Brad. *The Max Muscle Plan,* 1st ed. Champaign, IL: Human Kinetics. 2012.

56. Schoenfeld, Brad. *The Max Muscle Plan,* 1st ed. Champaign, IL: Human Kinetics. 2012.

About the Author

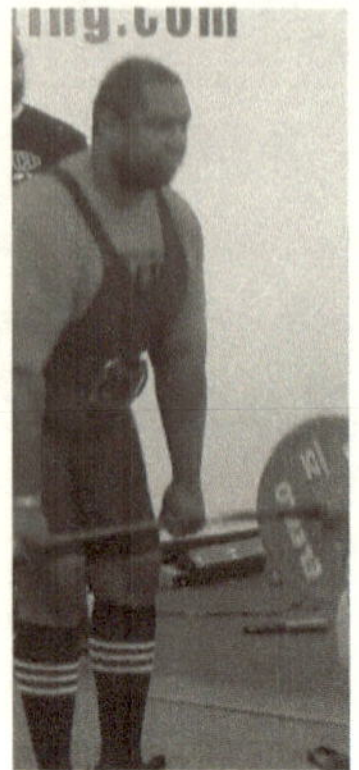

Phillip Germany II is an entrepreneur, trainer, and engineer and founder of Natural Strength and Fitness, a strength and wellness company that specializes in training people over 40. You can find more information at naturalstrengthandfitness.com.